Practical Yoga for Everyone

HOWARD MURPHET

Orient Longman

ORIENT LONGMAN LIMITED

Registered Office
3-6-272 Himayatnagar, Hyderabad 500 029 (A.P.), India

Other Offices
Bangalore / Bhopal / Bhubaneshwar / Chandigarh / Chennai
Ernakulam / Guwahati / Hyderabad / Jaipur / Kolkata
Lucknow / Mumbai / New Delhi / Patna

ISBN 81 250 0970 1

Typeset by
OSDATA
Hyderabad 500 029

Printed in India at
Isvarya Graphics
Hyderabad 500 004

Published by
Orient Longman Limited
3-6-272 Himayatnagar
Hyderabad 500 029

Contents

Foreword

This book was first published by Oldbourne Books of London in 1964, under the title *Yoga for Busy People*. When I was living in India a few years later, Oldbourne Books had disappeared. Presumably it had been reabsorbed into Beaverbrook Press from which it had originally come. So, although the first edition was a sell-out, there was no possibility of any new edition of this book. As I was still living in India, I offered the book to Orient Longman of India. I was very pleased when they accepted it and published it in 1971. It was published as a paperback for sale in India, Sri Lanka, South-east Asia and Africa. It continued to sell in those countries for over twenty years. Then in the year 1992, the publishers informed me that they would like to give the book what they called a facelift. By this I understood that they meant a volume of more substantial and attractive appearance. For the new book they asked me to make whatever revisions I felt were necessary. I was quite happy to do this because I felt that the book had proved its worth by being still alive and active some thirty years after I had first written it in 1963. I rewrote the first chapter which seemed inadequate. i made necessary changes in other chapters too. After years of study of yoga philosophy under various teachers in India, I felt that a postscript to the book was called for in order to bring the subject of the popular *Hatha Yoga* into a better perspective. I feel that this volume on practical yoga will prove of real value to the growing number of people throughout the world who are seeking a guide into this ancient but ever modern science and art of meaningful living.

This book is dedicated
to my wife Iris
in deep appreciation
of her constant help
and encouragement
in its production

CHAPTER ONE

Approach to Yoga

Heaven Lies Within Us is the title that Theos Bernard gave to his book on yoga. 'The kingdom of heaven is within you', stated the great yogi, Jesus of Nazareth. Yes, this is indeed the great truth, but the question is how do we bring that inner kingdom of happiness into manifestation in our daily lives.

But before we discuss that secret let us first clear away some popular misconceptions about yoga. It is not, for instance, an orthodox religion like Christianity, Islam or Buddhism. You can belong to any religion or no religion at all and still be a yogi. Neither is it a philosophy, although there is much philosophy in it. It is not an ascetic cult that denies all joys of living. On the contrary it brings much joy and meaning to life. It is not dangerous to practice yoga, any more than it is dangerous to eat or drink or play tennis. Most human activities are dangerous if carried to excess; few if practised in sensible moderation. The same is true of yoga.

We will gain a better understanding of what yoga is if we look for a moment at its origins. It was born long ago in ancient India and has developed through the centuries to the present age. When, over two centuries ago, the British established their trade stations in India and began to take some interest in the country, they came in contact with an ancient sacred literature written in Sanskrit. This is a language related to Latin and Greek, only, as one scholar put it, 'more perfect than Greek and more copious than Latin'. The root of the word Yoga is the Sanskrit verb *'yuj'* which means to *unite*. In Sanskrit literature scholars found references to yoga, which means 'union' or 'integration'. So yoga means to to unite something that is in a state of separation. It was apparently already well-known and practised at the time the books were written, thousands of years earlier. Some of our English words which have grown out of the same root are *join, junction, union,* and many other such words.

In the India around them, the British found men still practising yoga; they found that everyone revered it as a pathway to wisdom. But yoga, they soon discovered, is not just something you study, as you study philosophy or logic or history. It is something you do. The secret and the method lie in a 'doing' and a 'knowing'. These are partners, each helping and promoting the other. Both are given in the science and art of yoga. But the main thing is the doing – the action combined with the knowledge and philosophy behind it. Out of this doing grows a deeper understanding, a greater wisdom – the knowing.

There are different kinds of yogas – *Rajah, Hatha, Karma, Jnana, Bhakti* and *Mantra*. These are all pathways to the same goal but they emphasise different methods of reaching it. Yet the essential features of all are common. *Rajah Yoga* emphasises mind training, but it also calls for body exercise. *Hatha Yoga* concentrates on the thorough training of the body and at the same time trains the mind. *Karma Yoga* works through action in this world without concern for worldly fruits of action. The motive is duty or service to humanity. But all the yogas strive for this same detachment. *Jnana Yoga* emphasises knowledge and true discrimination; *Bhakti Yoga* devotion to a spiritual leader, and *Mantra Yoga* to the science of sound vibrations. Yet all yogas employ these instruments to some degree. While most Sanskrit works deal with the so called 'high yogas' i.e., *Karma, Jnana, Bhakti* and *Mantra* yogas, they do reveal some treasures of *Hatha Yoga*. If we liken yoga philosophy to a tree, we could say that *Hatha Yoga* forms the roots and the trunk. Continuing upward from the trunk and forming one of the main branches of the tree is *Rajah Yoga*. *Rajah Yoga* is closely intermeshed with *Hatha Yoga* in the trunk and is the yoga that concerns itself with the control and purification of the mind and emotions. In fact, *Hatha Yoga* leads into *Rajah Yoga*. There are four other main branches of the tree that reach upward from the trunk towards the blue vault of the sky that symbolises the heaven of man's aspirations. More will be said about these four branches of the great Yoga tree in the *Postscript* of this book. But, if and when the student of yoga finds himself in one of the higher branches, he should never neglect the trunk that supported him in his upward climb. In other words, whatever yoga you are following, however far you are up the leafy branch, you should remember to keep in good condition the trunk that supports it. No branch can continue to grow in strength without the supporting trunk and roots. So whatever level of yoga the aspirant may have reached, he should continue to practise in some degree the *Hatha Yoga* as taught in this book.

These different pathways are there to suit people of different types and temperaments. There are several intermediate unions to be achieved through the practise of yoga and a final union is its end and aim. You will have achieved at least some of these intermediate unions by the time you have learned and practised the physical and mental exercises given later in this book. All the pathways meet at the pinnacle of the mountain where ultimate union is achieved. What then is this union at which all yoga aims?

Man, we all agree, is a mysterious creature. He is made up of many elements – his body, his thinking mind, his feelings and desires, his ideals and conscience – to mention a few. Many of these elements are frequently at war with one another. We are a battleground for our urges, wishes, repressions and so on. Though we have probably never met one, we can imagine an ideal, perfected person in whom all these warring elements are united under the command of the Will. This person would, as a result, have perfect physical health, great courage, complete confidence and immense power. But, of course the Will that commands all the little selves must be an enlightened Will; otherwise the result may be a Black Magician who uses his great knowledge and power in a selfish, egocentric way, bringing suffering on his fellow men.

The ancient Indian sages, the yogis, believed – and mystics of all ages agree – that man has within him the potentiality of the Enlightened Selfless Will. The potentiality is the Divine spark. When it is fanned into a flame, the lower selves submit before the infinite wisdom. Man's Will identifies itself with the Divine Will.

This then is the high and ultimate purpose of yoga – to teach man to integrate himself, so that he feels complete union within himself, with the whole universe and with his Creator. This is all very fine, you might say, for ancient India and the other Asian countries to which yoga has spread. There was a type of social order in those places and times that allowed certain men to spend their whole lives in the development and practice of yoga. But what about us in the busy democratic, industrialised West – to what extent can we practise yoga and what benefits can we expect?

Yoga percolated very gradually to the Western world. A few Europeans like Indra Devi, a Russian by birth, who studied yoga from various teachers in India, and Michael Volin who learnt it from her, opened schools. Some Asians came West to lecture and teach yoga. Generally the yoga that was taught was *Hatha Yoga* – the approach through body training. This seems to have the greatest appeal to European thought. Today there is a *Hatha Yoga* school in most of the capitals of European countries and in some of the larger cities of USA, Australia, Canada and South Africa.

Traditionally, instruction in *Hatha Yoga*, which this book is all about, was given in an ashram by a dedicated guru to one or a small number of equally dedicated pupils. The pupils lived at the ashram so that the guru could direct their life in all its aspects. With the changing trends and values this kind of school has given rise to what is called the modern type of yoga school founded in Western countries and also now in India. Pupils go along to these types of schools for about an hour's instruction 2-3 times a week.

In the former type there is a greater devotion to what is called the yoga way of life as the instruction is more concentrated, there is close supervision by the guru of the disciple's diet and habits; yoga techniques – often strenuous – for inner cleanliness are taught and practised. The aim is to reach the ultimate state of union and integration in a few years or within one's lifetime.

In the latter type only important physical exercises, postures, breathing techniques and some mental exercises are taught. Hints are given about diet, hygiene, abstentions and self-discipline. But the pupil remains responsible for the conduct of his own life. Superficially, these schools may appear to be physical culture schools under another name.

I, myself, have been through several physical culture schools – civilian courses for teachers and training centres in the Services. Some of them aim to keep you fit, and up to a point, are successful. Some aim to develop large muscles, or spectacular skill in gymnastics. And if you work hard enough, they succeed. But their methods can be rather drastic; sometimes they drain energy rather than supply it. They have been known to stiffen joints, build muscle-bound bodies, and strain the heart. *Hatha Yoga's* objectives and methods are different. All its movements are smooth and graceful; there is a balance between tension and relaxation; physical movement is integrated with the right mental and emotional attitudes and with correct yogic breathing. The exercises do not drain energy but release extra energy to revitalise the body. The aim is not to build big muscles, win trophies or put up a spectacular display; it is to stabilise the forces in the body – uniting the *Ha,* that is the 'Sun', or the positive force with the *Tha,* meaning the 'Moon' or the negative force. While there are several important differences between ordinary physical culture and *Hatha Yoga* the main difference is that in yoga there is a conscious control and direction of *prana* which may also be called vital cosmic energy. This *prana* is in the body and moves in the body, whether you are aware of it or not. The universe itself is composed of this *prana* or cosmic energy. The movement and control of supplies of such energy comes under the *Atmic* or the highest human Will. While we could not do anything or even exist without the movement of this *prana,* the Will is like a supercharger that can increase the flow of *prana* to all parts of the body and to any particular part. The Will is the impelling force while the carrier of *prana* is the conscious mind. In brief wherever the conscious mind goes, *prana* goes. During my earliest lessons in yoga I gained the impression that breath carries the *prana.* I know now that although breath does play an important part, it is the conscious intention that sends the *prana.* 'The regulation of prana brings happiness – both worldly and spiritual,' states the great sage Vasishta in his revered authoritative work *Yoga Vasishta.* More will be said about this important subject in the following chapters.

The practical objectives of the modern yoga schools are :

1. to improve physical health towards ultimate perfection and to delay ageing;
2. to bring you to the right physical weight - neither too fat nor too thin;
3. to tap your inner reservoir of energy, thus continually revitalising the body;
4. to teach true relaxation and correct breathing and
5. to integrate the warring forces of the body and mind and develop an inner strength, so that you grow in poise, serenity and wisdom.

I have seen yoga do all of these things and anyone can test it for himself. All he needs is sufficient determination and faith to carry him on until he begins to feel some good effects – which will not be too long.

Perhaps it will help the reader to understand the aims and achievements of yoga if I relate something of my own experience. My aim in joining a modern school of yoga was to counter increasing flabbiness and to gain some measure of fitness. Of course I could have joined a physical culture class but the word yoga always appealed to me because, for some deeply subconscious reason, it suggested some mysterious depth and meaning below the surface. But all I was seeking at that time of my life in my late forties was a return to good health and fitness. The school I joined then, in the mid fifties, was, I think, the only one of its kind in New South Wales and probably in Australia too. It was known as the Sydney Yoga School and was conducted by Michael Volin, a Russian by birth.

Standing before his class of men and women of all ages, Michael Volin was an inspiration towards that I wanted to achieve. He was the personification of physical fitness with his perfectly sculptured body glowing with vital health and well-being. A feeling of calmness and tranquillity surrounded him.

This was an evening school and I found that most of the students went there at least two evenings a week and if possible, three. The class instruction in exercises, yoga postures, breath control and *pranayama* would go on for about forty-five minutes and then Volin would help and guide individual students who were attempting some of the more advanced postures. While talking to some yoga students, both male and female, I found that most of them had come initially, as I had myself, for such practical reasons as gaining better health, losing weight or gaining greater control of their emotional lives. But the most interesting fact was that when these aims were beginning to be achieved, they, like me, began showing an interest in yoga philosophy. The influence of the physical and mental exercises of *Hatha Yoga* seems to lead in some strange way to a yearning for a knowledge of yoga's ocean depths. A more important thing happened to me during those years at the Sydney Yoga School. It was there that I met my future wife, Iris, who was pupil at that school. In later years, after we had left Australia, we managed to have some lessons from a famous *Hatha Yoga* teacher in an ashram on the banks of the Ganges in India. While styles of presentation vary a little, as might be expected from teacher to teacher, fundamentally the instruction given by all is the same.

This fundamental instruction, along with details of procedures, controls and all necessary warnings, is presented in this book. If the directions and warnings given here are followed faithfully, particularly in regard to the time spent in postures and holding breath, known as *kumbhakas*, there is no danger whatsoever from yoga practice. On the contrary there is immeasurable benefit.

My wife, while a young student nurse, had an ice-skating accident where she fell backward on someone's upturned skate. This resulted in a cracked vertebra in the lumbar region of her spine. Tuberculosis bacteria entered the crack and began to eat away the bone. This was in the days when young British nurses were given a tough training and discouraged from mentioning their aches and pains. The trouble was not properly diagnosed until the germs had almost eaten away several of the vertebrae

The region of the spine was in a dangerously thin and delicate state – ready to snap at any moment, which would mean death or turn her into a permanent invalid.

The result was that she had to spend a whole year in bed immobilised on her back or stomach. A length of bone was cut from the tibia of her leg and grafted onto her spine to strengthen the weak region. The operation was successful, but the spine was stiff where there was the length of continuous bone instead of jointed vertebrae. The whole treatment took two years at the end of which she was able to move about and do light work but was told that she must always be careful, must never do heavy work or indulge in sports and recreations that she loved so much.

When I first met her, she was one of the star pupils at the *Hatha yoga* school, giving demonstration on the public platform and on television. Many of the demonstration postures called for a strength and flexibility of the spine well beyond the average. The yoga training had given her that remarkable strength and flexibility within a couple of years. Apart from reaching a high standard in yoga postures, she was able to resume her profession as a nurse – which often involved heavy lifting and carrying – and enjoy any sports and recreations that appealed to her. Hers is a case where the benefits of yoga seem almost miraculous.

Less dramatically, I have seen people cured of insomnia, asthma, nervous dyspepsia, and other psychosomatic troubles. I have seen them take inches off their waistlines and develop lithe and supple bodies. I have seen them grow self-controlled, confident and serene.

Patanjali, the great Indian sage who wrote the Yoga Sutras at around 300 BC, says, 'You must control the flow of ideas in your mind. If you can you will be your own true man, but if not you will be the pitiful victim of circumstance.'

This control of ideas and emotions often has great practical value. One winter day on the east coast of Australia, a teacher from the East went to take a dip in the Pacific. He did not know of the wild, powerful currents that are sometimes born out of winds and weather along that coast.

He dived off a flat rock into the sea and immediately found himself in the iron-handed grip of such a current which carried him rapidly out to sea. Instincts lead one to struggle violently against such a fate or to panic. But having tested the power of the current, the yogi knew that struggle was useless; it would merely squander his strength and he would drown. Relaxing and keeping completely calm, he let himself go with the current. He knew that its strength would peter out somewhere, and he hoped that from that point he would be able to swim back to land. He floated on his back, and elevated his consciousness until he seemed to be floating in the sky above the ragged scraps of cloud; he scarcely noticed the icy current that was carrying him out of sight of the Australian coast.

About two hours later he found himself not far off a sandy beach. The current had taken him in a great semi-circle and brought him back to the coast further north. Now its strength was spent, and he swam ashore.

An ordinary mortal would have suffered at least a chill and shock if nothing worse, but the same evening I saw the yogi instructing his group of students as if nothing had occurred. Yet if he had not controlled the inner currents of his body and mind, he would have been a victim to that vicious winter 'rip' – as the Australians call these spasmodic ocean currents.

SOME PRELIMINARY PRACTICAL POINTERS

There are several important practical questions that should be answered for those aspirants intending to practice the popular *Hatha Yoga* as described in the following chapters. One question is:

Who can do yoga?

The answer to this question is given in the ancient classic of *Hatha Yoga*, the *Hatha Yoga Pradipika* written in the distant past by a yoga guru named Swatmarama Swami. He states definitely and clearly that *Hatha Yoga* can be done by all people of both the sexes – adults of any age and also children and by both the healthy and the sick. I would like to qualify this by saying that anybody with a serious constitutional illness such as a weak heart should be very careful and circumspect in the way they practice. They should, no doubt, get medical advice before beginning. On the other hand, most medical authories do not understand the value of yoga when practised in a limited way. A perfect example of this is the case of my wife about whom you have already read earlier in this chapter. The younger you start yoga the better, of course, but I have known people begin at the age of seventy, and gain considerable benefit to health. I knew a business executive who learned to stand on his head at the age of 64. Although so near retiring age, he grew visible younger looking from the yoga exercises.

But can the busy millions of the modern world fit yoga practice into their waking hours? Many millions of my acquaintance have found that the busier they are, the more they need yoga. It enables them to relax quickly and fully enjoy their leisure after the long hours of hard grind.

Furthermore, by revitalising and renewing them, it enables them to get through more work in less time, and to labour longer hours without getting overfatigued.

Nancy Phelan, whom I knew as a yoga student in Australia, was a very busy woman indeed. In addition to normal duties as a housewife, she was taking care of an invalid father, writing books and broadcasting. Her average working day was twelve and a half hours. She could not, she said, have managed to get through all this without the revitalising yoga session. Later, she started conducting yoga classes as well, to add to her other activities and has, recently published a book on the subject.

Yet another busy writer who took up yoga to help her out is the novelist Freda Bromhead. She works hard at an office all day and writes in her 'spare time'. So, she would not seem to have too much time for anything else. But she decided that if she was going to have the vitality and endurance, the resilience and balanced relaxation to fit her writing into her other demanding activities, she must have lessons in yoga to fortify her. She now finds that yoga makes her the master of her mind, nerves, and the vital force of the body. It enables her to conserve and concentrate her energies and efforts to the purpose in view, without undue strain and nervous depletion.

Should a person start these practices without a personal instructor?

Do not be afraid to begin on your own if the instructions given here are carefully followed. The well-known American yogi, Theos Bernard, for example, began without a personal supervisor and with no textbook of instruction to guide him. All he had was, words of advice and directions given to him by a teacher who came on a visit, after which Bernard was left to his own resources. Some years after he had made good progress on his own a personal guru came into his life. This is in keeping with the well-known occult law, which says, 'When the pupil is ready, the guru will appear.'

So, begin alone or with a like-minded friend. Follow the instructions given here carefully and when you have advanced to the point where you need a personal teacher, one will come into your life.

When and where to do yoga?

The answer to the first part of the question is, to practise whenever it is convenient provided it is at least three hours after a meal. Otherwise, any time of the day or evening is suitable. Before breakfast is a good time to do some breathing and warming-up exercises, but many people find their joints too stiff so early in the morning for the majority of the postures.

The place to practice should be a quiet room where you are alone. There should be plenty of fresh air in the room; yet it is better to practise indoors than outdoors. If practising outdoors, you will find it easier to do the exercises and postures in the shade rather than in hot sunshine. Yoga practice should be as private as possible. Like meditation, it is something between you and a Higher Power. Its aim is to decrease, not increase your ego and pride. Trained yogis can sit cross-legged or stand on their heads in a busy market place, without being in the slightest degree distracted by the noise and commotion. They are completely withdrawn and detached from their surroundings. But beginners should choose some quiet, secluded place either alone or with other yoga students, for their yoga sessions.

Many of the special exercises given for busy people can be performed at odd times and in all kinds of places – in buses, trains, cars, in office or factory, or while walking from one place to another.

What to wear?

The clothes you wear for yoga must of course be suitable for the climate and season. Whatever they are, they should be loose-fitting and never tight enough to restrict movement. The aim is to wear as little as possible, giving the body full freedom of movement. In warm climates, men usually wear nothing but a pair of swimming trunks, while women wear bathing or sun suits. If it is too cold for trunks or short, other possibilities are loose-fitting slacks and shirt, track suits and leotards. It is a good idea to have handy a little covering of some kind to put over the body while lying still in a deeply-relaxed pose. You should have a folded blanket or rug on the floor or perhaps a mat on dry, level ground, which make a good base on which to perform the sitting, standing or lying postures.

How long?

Beginners, who are working without a teacher, should not spend more than forty-five minutes to an hour in a session of yoga exercises. Of course, devotees of the traditional schools sometimes spend that much time in one posture alone. But students leading the life of today's world must avoid any excess of zeal. The length of time to be spent in each posture will be indicated with the instruction for its execution.

Attitude

Although the exercise are a form of self-discipline, there should be pleasure in the performance as well as in the final fruits. If you enjoy every movement and posture thoroughly, the benefit will be increased greatly. Remember that slow movement – not speed or jerkiness – is the aim. Never force or strain muscles in order to reach a certain position. Do not think of how a posture looks to someone else, but of the good it is doing you. Keep the mind calm throughout.

Hatha Yoga is primarily a training of the body but body and mind are so closely interwoven and integrated that it inevitable changes the mind also. While character training and development come as a by-product of both *Hatha* and *Rajah Yoga*, they also call for a firm basis of moral and ethical behaviour in the student at the beginning. For this purpose, some of the old textbooks set out rules and regulations for self-control and ritualistic practices. For the modern student, such a list of do's and don'ts may not have much meaning, so in place of them I will give here Sai Baba's five Pillars of Wisdom for what he calls Education in Human Values. These may also be called guidelines of behaviour or beacons to guide the individual's ship of life.

1. The first of these is *Truth.* This not only means aiming to find the deepest truth but living always by Truth as we know it. A good yogi will never deviate from the Truth for any selfish reason.
2. The second pillar of wisdom is *Universal Love.* This means, the yogi must aim to love and feel at one not only with all human beings, but with all life. As the student directs his footsteps more and more by this guideline he will begin to perceive the Divinity in all being which is the basis of the feeling of unity or universal love.
3. The shining pillar of wisdom called *Peace* is the third. The student strives to attain true peace within himself and his yoga practice will help him in this. Inner peace leads naturally to outer peace in the family, in the community and indeed in the world.
4. A fourth guiding light for the student is *Non-violence.* Again this must begin in one's mind and heart. There must be no violent, harmful or aggressive thoughts towards others. It follows as night follows day that if there is no violence in the mind or the heart there will be none in words or actions. You will see how close this principle of behaviour is to universal love and peace, all of which belong to the deep spiritual truth of life.

5. When these four guidelines are followed they naturally lead to the fifth pillar of wisdom in human behaviour, called *dharma* in Sanskrit. We can translate it as *right-living* in English.

Every yoga student being a unique individual will live according to the guidelines in his own special way and make his unique contribution to their development. All the authorities on yoga, both ancient and modern, state from experience and observation that practical *Hatha Yoga* will bring radiant health, vigour and vitality by balancing and harmonising the positive and negative forces between the body and mind while adding years to the life of the practitioner. In fact, yoga says that the length of life should not be three score years and ten but a hundred and fifty years. But whether you want more years in your life or not, you will certainly want more life in your years. The faithful and constant practice of yoga as described in the following chapter will undoubtedly enrich the years of your life.

CHAPTER TWO

How to Relax in Depth

At some time every man will ask himself this question: 'What do I mean when I use the word "I"? What am I?' Even primitive man felt instinctively, and believed, that he was more than his body. Modern man tends to identify himself with the part that thinks and feels – the part that is usually called the 'mind'. But when he is trying to control it, and is somehow standing aside from it, he begins to realise that it cannot be his whole essential self. If 'mind' is something that he calls 'his', something that he attempts to control and use, how can it be him, himself?

Both body and mind are best thought of as instruments, pieces of equipment, vehicles, if you like, of the Real Self. But, like a car with the brakes gone, they often take control, and run away with the driver.

That is what is happening to most of the people most of the time. They are being carried here, there, and everywhere by their emotions, instincts and desires. To control the body and mind, we must first learn how closely, how subtly, they work together.

The mind, though non-physical, is expressed through many physical centres – not only through the brain, but all the nerve channels that go to every part of the body. Every cell has a degree of consciousness of its own; it can respond to the mind, and the mind can respond to it.

As an example of this, if a man is told something that pleases his mind his face will light up, and he may leap to his feet. Should it be bad news that he hears, his body will droop. Conversely, a particular mental state can be created by a bodily posture. Lift the corners of your mouth in the expression of a smile, for instance, and you will feel cheerful. Dance a joyous jig, and any clouds of depression will evaporate. The rhythms of a tribal war-dance build up martial feelings in the warrior's mind.

In brain-washing techniques severe physical suffering is used to wash the mental slate clean.

In a more subtle and quiet way this interaction between body and mind is going on all the time. On the one hand, the events of the body – the things you eat, the physical exercises you do, the air you breathe – affect your thoughts, your feelings, and your character. Dr Joseph Bancroft of Cambridge University said that when the brain gets insufficient oxygen, there is a tendency to impatience and irritability. On the other hand, the mental states and emotions of everyday life – the joys and sorrows, love and hatred are constantly working on your biochemistry – changing your physical vehicle for good or ill.

Too much anxiety and nervous tension can change your body functioning to the extent of causing sickness. Medical science admits this in the case of psychosomatic diseases, such as migraine, indigestion, stomach ulcers, certain heart troubles and types of asthma. But if we could penetrate deeply enough, we would probably find mental causes at the base of many other physical ailments.

During the last century, the tempo of life has been increasing rapidly. Modern man does much more and goes much further in a given time than his forefathers would have dreamed possible – or even desirable. In fact *speed* in all phases of life is mounting to a frightening crescendo.

The dizzy end of this way of living is shown in the story of the man who went to a psychiatrist and said: 'Doctor, my mind is like a spinning top. Everything flies straight off it. I can't remember a thing the moment it's happened.'

'And how long has this been going on?' asked the psychiatrist.

To which the patient replied, 'How long has what been going on?'

In this Nuclear Age, there is also, added to the growing pressure of speed, the fear of annihilation. And after the great annihilating explosion, what then? The scientific spirit has not only brought the engines of speed, but also the enquiring mind that doubts – or rejects outright – the old teachings about a hereafter. As far as he can prove scientifically, man has only this earth life – and he thinks, under the circumstances, probably not much of that. Life seems devoid of ultimate meaning; man snatches greedily, despairingly at what the moment offers, as he races towards the brink of Nothingness.

The evolution of life on earth, from the simplest forms to the complex creature called man, has depended on the ability of the life force to adapt itself to new conditions. When there is a drastic change, any form of life that fails to make the necessary adjustments goes to the wall; yet the powerful principle of life has always gone on, unfolding itself into new patterns.

Man has now to adjust himself to conditions drastically different from the natural environment in which he was slowly evolved. And as subconscious tensions are multiplying at a high rate, the adjustments must be made swiftly.

Fortunately he does not have to rely on the hidden forces of Nature for this. He has reached the level of development where he can use his individual consciousness, his will, and any know-how that he may have.

The scientific technique evolved by the ancient yogis makes use of the close inter-relationship between the body and mind, in order to bring both these vehicles under complete control of the Will. The old sages were not so concerned with immediate health aims as the ultimate purpose of 'stilling' the mind in order to go beyond it into a higher consciousness. But, whatever long term hopes we ourselves may cherish, we can use their know-how to bring the mind and body under complete control for the immediate purpose of relaxing, renewing, and revitalising our vehicles.

In this way we will learn to strengthen our mechanisms and adjust them to the unnatural conditions and anxieties of the industrialised world.

The ability to calm and control subconscious fears that rage through the nerves at the imminence of pain and danger is a great step forward. But yogis of long experience go further. They are able to detach the mind from all concerns of body sensations, so that even major surgical operations can be performed on them without anaesthetics. Yogananda writing about the appendix operation performed on Mahatma Gandhi, for which he had refused to have anaesthetics says that Mahatma Gandhi 'chatted cheerfully with his disciples throughout the operation, his infectious smile revealing his unawareness of pain.'

Hatha Yoga relaxation operates on the principle that the mind can be more easily and profoundly reached through the body than vice versa. Certain yoga postures— such as the cross-legged ones to be explained later—have in themselves a calming effect on the mind. But in the relaxation posture, the conscious Will is used to relax the body bit by bit. When the body is perfectly relaxed, the mind cannot be otherwise. Conversely, when the mind is truly relaxed, there can be no tensions in the body.

Here are two preliminary relaxation exercises that can be performed either in succession as shown, or singly at different times. Before beginning, remain quiet for a few minutes, try to empty the mind of all tension, and throughout the exercise think of nothing but the bodily sensations created.

Exercise 1

Standing with the feet apart, raise the arms in front of the body, and hold them for a moment parallel with the floor. Now suddenly withdraw all the nervous energy from the arms, and let them fall to the sides. At the same time drop the head loosely forward onto the chest. Let the arms hang slackly, and relax the neck and face. Breathe naturally. Repeat the exercise about a dozen times. Remember, stance and movements must be free and easy – none of the old ramrod stiffness loved by the sergeant-major!

Exercise 2 *[Fig. 1]*

Standing in the same manner with feet apart, drop the head forward onto the chest, and – as a continuation of the same movement – let the whole trunk go forward from the waist, bending so that the arms hang loosely towards the floor. Don't be rigid. Be floppy. Shake the arms and face muscles – getting rid of all the tensions.

Then come up to the starting position, and repeat the exercise until the whole upper part of the body feels relaxed and glowing.

Breathe naturally throughout. Let yourself really go, and thoroughly enjoy it.

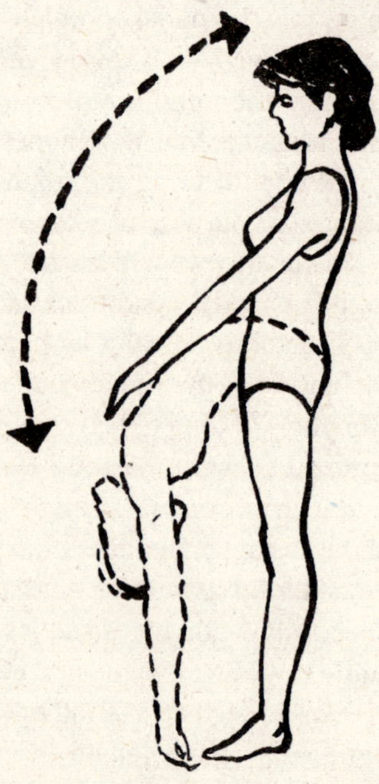

Fig. 1

The Relaxation Posture *[Fig. 2]*

In Sanskrit this was called the *Savasana,* which means 'Dead-body posture'. At first sight it appears easy to play the dead body, but to do it well, to gain the full happy effect, requires practice and patience.

Preparation

Spread your folded blanket on the hard floor and lie down flat on your back, with arms loosely by your sides, in the most comfortable position. Breathe naturally.

Phase I

Remembering that tension is something the mind can perceive in the muscles, begin to relax the parts of the body. Start with the toes. Send your conscious attention right into the part and tell it to relax. Say mentally, 'My toes are relaxing'; 'My feet are relaxing', 'My ankles are relaxing', 'Now they are completely relaxed', and so on for the rest of the body. Let the mind linger in the part; locate even the slightest tension there and release it.

Following this method, relax your legs, hands, arms, trunks, neck, face and head. For a thorough job it is better, at first, to divide some of these major sections into smaller parts. In the face, for example, concentrate separately on the eyes, the lips, the cheeks. Other important parts to work on specially for deep relaxation are the tongue, vocal cords, and the jaws – so that the mouth sags open.

Having been once or twice through your body in this way, let the mind rove quietly through again, searching out any tensions that have lingered or crept back. If any of these prove hard to draw away, consciously *tense* the part concerned, and then let go and relax it. This pre-tension before

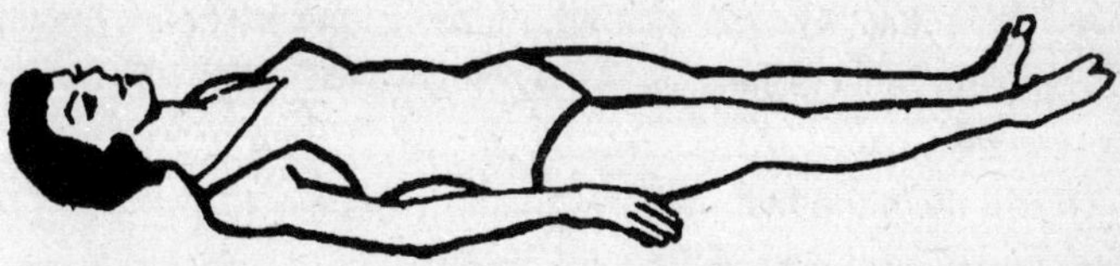

Fig. 2

relaxation can be a great help. Another useful trick is to picture the tension as a bubble, and imagine it rising to the surface and vanishing – just as bubbles move out of a liquid.

While you relax, imagine yourself becoming so heavy that you could sink through the floor. Say mentally a number of times—'I am getting heavy - very heavy - and relaxed.'

Phase 2

When you feel so heavy that you could sink down through the earth, start to watch your breathing. Breathe very deeply so that your stomach rises and falls slowly and rhythmically. Feel that the sensation of heaviness is changing to a wonderful lightness. With each breathe you take, imagine yourself growing more and more like a floating cloud.

Your eyes are shut, and if you concentrate on the thought of becoming as light as vapour, you will actually have the illusion of floating, because when all tensions have gone, you do not feel your body at all.

Now you must keep the mind as still as possible. One way to do this is to observe the little figures and shapes that appear behind your closed eyelids. Concentrate on them so that there is no room for other thoughts in the focus of consciousness. Thoughts will hover around the fringe. Don't fight or invite them; just let them float idly by. Your aim is complete mental stillness, and if you achieve this, even for a moment, you will gain a great refreshment.

Conclusion

Put your arms over your head; stretch your whole body, yawn and gently come to a sitting position. Yawn and stretch again, then get slowly to your feet. Never jump up quickly.

Some Aids to Relaxing Muscles and Mind

1. Imagine that you are slowly immersing your muscles in warm water.
2. Imagine that you have fallen asleep on a soft green sward by the sea. You are just regaining consciousness, with the warm sun on your face, and the song of the waves in your ears.
3. As you exhale imagine that all your tensions are being drawn away from your inner organs, as an outgoing wave sucks away the sand and seaweed.
4. To still the mind focus the eyes on a small object several feet beyond the end of your nose. Alternatively, close the eyes and look at a simple image, such as a rose or a ripe peach—or just an imaginary point—in this position. Your eyes will be turned slightly inwards.

When and How Often to do the Relaxation Posture.

This posture can be done at any time that is convenient and the student can stay in the posture as long as he is comfortable and has the time. Of course, if he stays too long, he will probably go to sleep. The thing to remember is that there is no danger in this posture but only benefits.

If you wish, the posture can be done in bed before going to sleep, but first remove the pillow. Beginners sometimes like to have a small, rolled pillow under the neck to tilt the head back. This can be helpful.

A hard floor is actually better than anything soft for relaxing on, and it's more enjoyable once you get used to the idea.

Some Benefits

In *Savasana (Fig. 2)* the circulation of the blood is in equilibrium, the blood pressure is lowered, and the work of the heart relieved. Within the nervous system there is rest and refreshment. Practice of the posture will tend to prevent and alleviate psychosomatic diseases. The posture is used by a psychiatrist of my acquaintance to cure insomnia. A person who learns to relax properly, at will, learns an important part of the formula for a happy, healthy life.

Quick Relaxers

The following should be used in spare minutes throughout the day. They will get you into the priceless habit of relaxing during those activities that tend to drive you relentlessly onward, whether it be in office, home or factory.

(a) Stand up and do Exercise 1 above (you may need to be alone for this.)

(b) While either sitting or standing, shake the hands and arms as a cat shakes a mouse. Feel them going loose and free.

(c) Standing, do likewise with the legs and feet. Shake the tensions out of them – one leg at a time, of course!

(d) Sitting, let the head fall forward on the chest. Let the arms droop, relax the face muscles, and rest. The boss may not like the look of this; but the truth is you will work twice as efficiently afterwards.

(e) Rest your elbows on the desk or table as you sit. Lean forward and cover your eyes with the palms of your hands. Keep out the light, but do not press against the eyeballs. Stay there a few minutes, breathing deeply and calming the mind. Think only of REST and PEACE. This is called palming.

Try to do one of these quick relaxers every hour throughout the day. Get into the habit. After a while you will find yourself observing your mind and body at intervals as they work. You will probably find your left hand clenched when your right hand is pounding something, for example, or your facial muscles tense because your brain is busy on a controversial matter.

This is largely because the subconscious mind, influenced by remnants of racial memories, has been sending out warning signals. It flashed, 'On guard' to that left hand, 'Action stations' to the facial muscles, for instance, and both of these were unnecessary because you did not have to flatten an enemy with your fist, or frighten him off with your facial expression.

Now as you learn to observe and remove these out-of-place, and out-of-date, muscular tensions, your actions will become more relaxed and controlled; you will save a great deal of vitality, and be more efficient in all you do.

As you advance in the yoga exercises and self-observation, your leisure, your rest – even your sleep – will be more beneficial; deep tensions, buried worries will be cleared out of the mental attics from which they were poisoning both mind and body.

CHAPTER THREE

Breathing and the Yoga Breath

Breathing is something that we have been doing automatically since the moment we were born. It is directed subconsciously, but can be brought under conscious control – as indeed can the heart-beat and other subconscious bodily activities.

When the actual process of breathing is analysed, it is found to be quite an intricate business. The lungs hang loosely in the chest, each in a separate compartment. Air is brought in by an expansion brought about through either of two methods – or preferably both combined. One, a sheet of muscular tissue, called the diaphragm, which divides the lung area from the abdomen, may be drawn downward. Or, two, other muscles may swing the ribs, which are hinged to the spine, outward and upward. When these two sets of respiratory muscles relax and recoil to their natural position, the air is expelled from the lungs.

The atmosphere is filled with dust and bacteria. To guard against these reaching the lungs, the nasal passages are lined with hair to act as screens, glands secrete sticky mucus, and microscopic hairs flail back and forth, sweeping the dust particles towards the throat. Swallowed, the debris will be harmless in the digestive tract. The millions of bacteria breathed into the nose are killed in the upper airways by a special germ-destroying enzyme contained in the mucous secretions. At the same time, as it passes along the passages, the air is warmed to the correct temperature and moistened to the right degree of humidity before it reaches the lungs. With the nasal corridors providing such a capable air-conditioning and filtering system, it is easy to see why you should breathe through the nose and not the mouth.

After its treatment in the nose, the air passes down the windpipe which divides like a tree-trunk into two stems, one going to the right lung and the other to the left. Each stem spreads into a network of branches which we call the bronchial tubes. The smallest tubes finally open into clusters of tiny air sacs. There are about 750 million of these, and like the leaves of a tree, they are planned to provide an entire surface area. In fact, it is estimated that the total wall area of the air sacs in your lungs would cover a plane surface of about 455 square feet (approx. 42.27 sq. m.).

This double-stemmed tree inside your chest, bringing in the vital elements from the outside world, is met by another tree from the heart. This consists of blood vessels that finally branch out into thousands of cobwebby capillaries. You can think of these as a fine foliage that clings to, and covers, the air leaves (the sacs) of the lung tree.

Blood, bearing the carbon dioxide and waste from the body, is pumped to these tiny capillaries, entering them as a blue black liquid. Their passageways are so narrow that the blood cells must pass along in single file. Yet all the blood cells of your body must march through these narrow capillaries in about three minutes for the necessary aeration. Through the gossamer-thin walls the blood gives up its heavy load of carbon dioxide, and takes on life-giving oxygen. Now the liquid is bright cherry-red as it leaves the capillaries and moves off to carry oxygen to the millions upon millions of cells throughout the human body.

The actual transporting is done by the red blood cells, of which there are about 250 million for every drop of blood. These carriers work so hard that their life span is only about thirty days. This means that, to replace them, twelve million blood cells must be produced every second.

The exchange of gases between the air tree and the blood tree goes on unceasingly day and night. Normally we take from 15 to 20 breaths a minute, and with each breath, we inhale about a pint (0.588 lit.) of air. *Resting* lungs hold six pints of air. So this means that only about one-sixth of the air in the lungs is changed with each breath. But through deep breathing or rapid breathing, or both, we can increase the intake of air by ten, or more, times.

The majority of people never exercise their lungs properly or use them to full capacity. They cramp them with poor postures and treat them to atmospheres that nature never intended. They breath in a shallow mechanical way, using only the upper part of the lungs, and seldom if ever, 'flush them out' by deep breathing in clear, fresh air.

Our urban life and sedentary occupations are partly to blame for this, but not entirely. I have seen farmers, who walked the fields, breathing God's own good air all their days, go down with bronchial asthma in what should have been the prime of their lives.

People who enjoy plenty of outdoor sports often suffer, nevertheless, from respiratory and chest troubles.

There is no doubt that correct deep breathing is one of the foundation stones of physical fitness and sound health. but yoga takes breathing a step further than this. There is a subtle but very real relationship between breath and mind – between breathing and thinking or feeling. There is something you may have learned from everyday experience. If you get excited, you begin to breath quickly. When you are nervous or apprehensive – perhaps before making a public speech – you can calm yourself down with a few slow deep breaths. If you are thinking too much, and can't get off to sleep, some steady deep breathing will slow the racing mind and get you in the right mental state for slumber.

Yoga techniques make use of this strange connection between breath and mind to gain a mastery over the mind – over its thoughts, desires, imaginings – through a system of breath-control exercises.

In this way the conscious manipulation of the breathing mechanism leads to better physical and mental health, first through better oxygenation of the blood, and secondly through control and unification of the conflicting psychic forces in mind and nerves. At the same time it leads to inner calmness and equanimity.

Apart from the physical and mental aspect of breathing, yogi sages have always taught that there is a subtle life-giving force available to us. It is in all created things – not only in the air we breathe, but the food we eat, and the liquids we drink. In Sanskrit, this basic life force was called '*prana*'.

Prana is not a thing that has been isolated and identified in the scientific research laboratories. But that does not mean it does not exist. There was a time when the great forces of electricity, radio waves, X-rays, and many others, were not known to science. But they all existed, and had existed since the beginning of time. There are doubtless many hidden forces still working in the universe that have so far eluded capture by the apparatus of the research scientists.

By its careful, exact and tireless efforts science is doing wonderful work for mankind. But we must not make the grave error of thinking that nothing exists unless its existence has been demonstrated and accepted by modern science. The search for precise truth, which we call science, has never stood still. It has always moved on— sometimes rapidly, sometimes slowly— discovering new things.

As the centuries passed, more and more knowledge was unearthed and documented for man's use, but great hidden depths of knowledge still lie untapped. We might say of the march of science what Tennyson said of 'experience' – that it is 'an arch wherethrough gleams that untravelled world whose margin fades forever and forever as I move'.

The great yogis proved the force of *prana* for themselves in the laboratory of life. They proved it by working what we might call miracles – curing diseases, building stupendous vitality, developing supernormal powers of strength, resistance, endurance, retaining youthful vigour, and living in robust health to incredible ages.

They teach that this vital energy is already working in you – it is your basic force – but that you can increase the quantity by becoming consciously aware of it, and opening yourself mentally to its flow.

Yoga exercises help you to do this, particularly the breathing exercises. As you breathe in, you should think of the great *pranic* current flowing into your body. When you exhale, the air – laden with carbon dioxide and other impurities – passes out, but the *prana* remains. You can think of it seeping right through you into every cell, bringing extra life, strength and perfect health.

If you do this, you will feel the benefits almost immediately, and will have no doubt that some extra force is at work – something that you can call upon and consciously direct within your own Being. Some yoga students have had startling results after just a few months of practising the conscious direction of *prana*; they have found that it could revitalise tired aching limbs, remove little irritating troubles and complaints, such as nerve pains, headache, sore throats and even cure instantly small burns that otherwise would have been painful for days.

It does not really matter how you name this undocumented, but very potent force. You may wish to call it 'auto-suggestion'. Under that label it has helped many thousands of people in the past. You may like to call it a 'psychic ray'; it will not be offended, and will work just as well for you under that name.

The ancient Chinese healers believed in a force they called Qi. This, they thought, operated along the nerve channels of the body, and by stimulating its flow, they cured many illnesses. Science has not detected and identified this force either, but it seems to be real enough. In the West, as well as in modern China, qualified medical men are making use of it through the technique of Acupuncture, to cure a long list of diseases. Qi may be a special, more limited, form of the great all-pervading creative force that the Indian sages called *prana*.

The Complete Yoga Breath *(Fig. 3)*

This full yoga breath should be used in all breathing exercises unless otherwise directed.

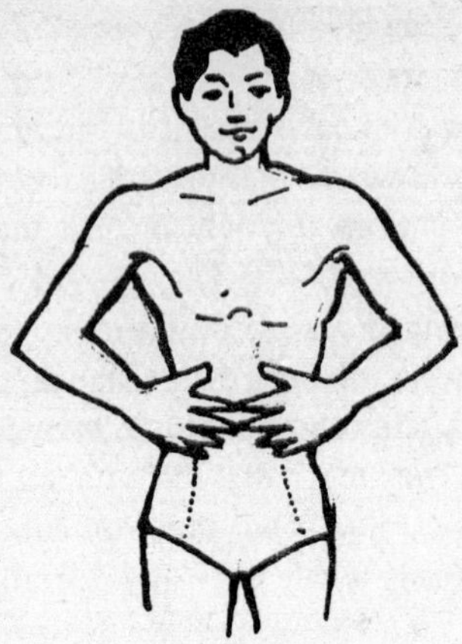

Fig. 3

Stand with feet apart or lie on your back in the relaxation posture. With hands open and palms inward, place them on the abdomen so that the thumbs are just below the floating ribs and the fingers of the two hands are meeting in front. Press the abdomen inwards and at the same time breathe out with a long slow breath. Clear as much air as possible from the lungs. This will be helped by grunting as you press with your hands.

Expand the abdomen so that it pushes the hands downward, forward and sideways. This means that your diaphragm is moving downward and the lower lungs are filling with air. If you are inhaling correctly, you will feel and hear the pressure of air at the back of the palate and throat. There should be no sniffing sensation or noise in the nostrils.

When you have expanded the abdomen as much as possible, transfer your attention to the middle part of the thorax. To help you do this, slide your hands upward over your lower ribs, and expand this part so that the air streams into the middle lungs. Finally, slide the hands onto the chest, and feel this arching outward as you draw all the air possible into the upper lungs. In this last phase, the abdomen will be drawn in a little to help the full expansion of the chest.

Viewed from the side of the body, the yoga breath appears like a slow wave forming in the abdomen and swelling upward to the chest. There must be a smooth transition from one phase of the breath to another.

Exhale by letting the air go out through the mouth like a gas escaping from a pricked ballon. At the same time drop the hands to the sides and relax.

Practice this basic yoga breath for several minutes in the fresh air before breakfast each day, and several other times during the day, until you can breathe into the diaphragm, and create the tidal wave upward to the chest, with ease. Remember, before inhaling you must first *empty* the lungs as far as possible. The full yoga breath is the foundation stone of all yoga breathing exercises, and the beginning of your transformation in health and personality.

Note: In many yoga breathing exercises the exhalation is not done quickly through the mouth as described above, but through the nose – easily and naturally, or else controlled to a certain tempo as directed for particular exercises.

CHAPTER FOUR

Transform Yourself Through Breath Control

An average human lifetime is about 500 million breaths. There is a yoga saying that each individual is allotted a certain number of breaths in his life span; if he takes them slowly, his life will be correspondingly longer. This is just another way of saying that deep, slow breathing prolongs our sojourn on earth.

It is certain that shallow breathing, in which most people indulge most of the time, does not aerate the blood properly. This means that purification and reconstruction throughout the body is not carried out fully and efficiently.

Many of the yoga breathing exercises involve not only the inhalation of a large volume of air, but the retention of the air in the lungs for a certain period. What are the effects of breath retention from a physiological point of view?

Lungs are never empty. After exhaling, you still have about 200 cubic centimetres of air spread throughout the bronchial tubes and sacs. But only the air in the sacs is able to exchange gases in the blood, because the walls of the bronchial tubes are too thick for gases to penetrate.

You take a breath, and fresh air highly charged with oxygen comes into the lungs. Now, it is the manner of arrival in the little air sacs that indicates the value of breath retention. Experiments have been made which show that the mixing of the new air with the static air in the sacs takes time. Furthermore, the fresh air enters in the form of a cone pointing into the centre of the sac, so that the old impure air, still lies in a layer around the walls until proper diffusion can take place. Unless the new air is retained in the sacs for the necessary length of time, diffusion will not take place properly, and the air lying close to the walls will remain too highly charged with carbon dioxide; the blood will not be able to secure its vital oxygen as readily and completely as it should. Breath retention, as taught in the yoga exercises, allows for perfect mixing of the airs in the little sacs, and this, of course, means efficient oxygenation of the blood.

DEVELOPMENT EXERCISES

The following breathing exercises are the foundation stones of *Hatha Yoga.* They develop the respiratory muscles, expand the chest and lungs, and strengthen the will power. This enables you to move on to more advanced breath control, or *pranayama* as it is called in oriental yoga. The exercises will also help you to breath correctly in the yoga postures, and this is extremely important.

A few general practical points to remember are : practise in a quiet, well-ventilated place; keep the mind and feelings calm and the face serene, think of *nothing* except the exercise. Open yourself to *prana* that flows in with each inhalation. As you breathe out, think that you are sending the impurities, fatigue, tensions away, but retaining *prana* within your body; it is bringing you perfect health, strength and vitality. Be quite convinced of this, know that it is happening, and it will indeed be so.

Routine 1

For this routine stand easily with feet apart, and the hands at the sides. Inhalation is through the nose and exhalation through the mouth.

(a) Take a full yoga breath. Slap the chest several times with both hands while holding the breath. Then breathe out and drop the hands.

(b) Take a full breath. Hold it while you raise your arms and extend them in front of you, parallel, relaxed, palms downward. Draw them back slowly until they are bent at the shoulders. Thrust them forward again, and then drop them to your sides as you exhale. (With more practice, you can draw the arms back slowly and shoot them forward twice, while holding a breath). Repeat the exercise once.

(c) Take a full yoga breath. Hold it while you raise your arms and place them in front of the chest, palms together in the gesture of prayer. Press the hands together, feeling the tension in arms and chest. Lower them while exhaling. Repeat the exercise once.

(d) (Fig. 4) Take a full yoga breath. Hold it while you bend to the right from the waist, at the same time swinging the arms sideways and upwards to touch each other over the head. Without pausing, swing the arms down to the sides again as you bring the trunk upright. Still retaining the breath,

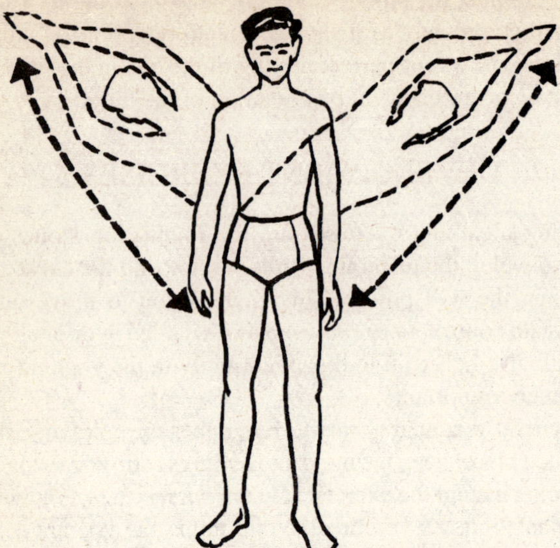

Fig. 4

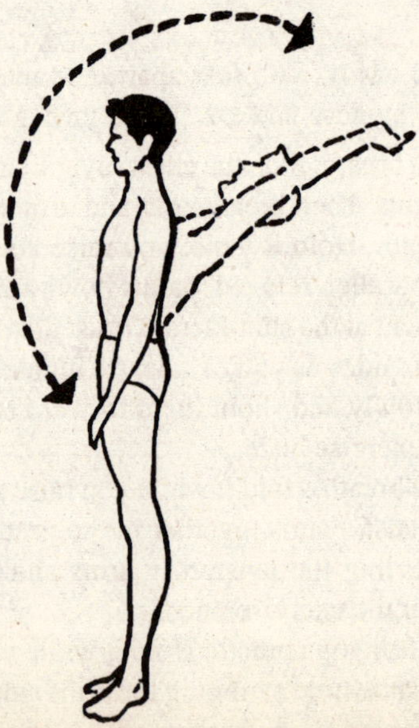

Fig. 5

repeat the movements to the left side. Then, as you finally bring the arms downward and straighten the trunk, let the breath go out. Repeat the exercise once.

(e) (Fig. 5) Take a full yoga breath. Hold it while you bend backward from the waist, swinging your arms forward and upward over your head as you bend back. Straighten up, bringing the arms forward and downward to the sides again. Repeat the movement, exhaling as you drop the arms the second time. Repeat the exercise once.

(f) Take a full yoga breath, and hold it. Swing your arms sideways and upward, linking them over the head. Turn the trunk to the right, as if you are trying to look behind you; feel the muscles stretching at the side of the abdomen. Do the same towards the left side. Then as you face forward again, lower the arms and exhale. Repeat the exercise once.

The whole routine will take less than three minutes.

Routine 2

Stand with the feet apart, knees slightly bent, shoulders sagging forward, head dropped on the chest. Relax the whole of the body, particularly the face. Breathe out completely.

Inhale through the nose with a double breath – a short quick breath followed by a long one. Fill the lungs fully from the diaphragm to the chest; at the same time tense the muscles of the body from toes to head, raising the arms forwards, and swinging them outwards to stretch sideways at shoulder level. Now with the lungs full, the body tense, and the arms stretched on either side, palms downward, bend the head back and turn the arms so that the palms face upward. Mentally count 1, 2, 3 at about the speed of seconds.

Next breathe out through the mouth with a double breath – a short one followed by a long complete exhalation. At the same time swing the arms forward, and drop them downward; relax the body; droop the head forwards, and assume the original loose, sagging posture. Repeat six times. Try to really let go and become increasingly relaxed after each exhalation, try to tone up the muscles by strong, positive tension with each inhalation.

This routine will also take you less than three minutes.

Routine 3

Stand with feet apart and hands at the sides. Both inhalation and exhalation are through the nose.

(a) Breathe deeply into the abdomen as you raise the arms sideways. When the hands come above the head, interlock the fingers, turn the palms

upward, and stretch the arms as far up as possible to form an arch above you. Look up at the backs of the interlocked hands. The lungs should now be completely full of air.

Hold the breath for a few seconds, then straighten the neck, and lower the arms slowly to the sides, breathing out through the nose in a long controlled breath.

(b) Inhale, raising the arms as in *(a)*. While looking upward, bend from the waist towards the right as far as possible, then towards the left. Finally lower the arms, and breathe out as before.

(c) This is the same as *(b)* except that you bend forward and backward from the waist, instead of sideways, while looking up at the hands. Exhale as before.

(d) (Fig. 6) The same as *(c)* except that, instead of bending backward and forward, you circle from the hips, first in a clockwise direction for one whole circle, then in an anticlockwise direction for one whole circle. Make the circles as large as you can with comfort.

If you find difficulty in holding your breath, do only one circle for each breath, until your will-power and muscle control improve. Exhale as before.

This routine will only take a couple of minutes.

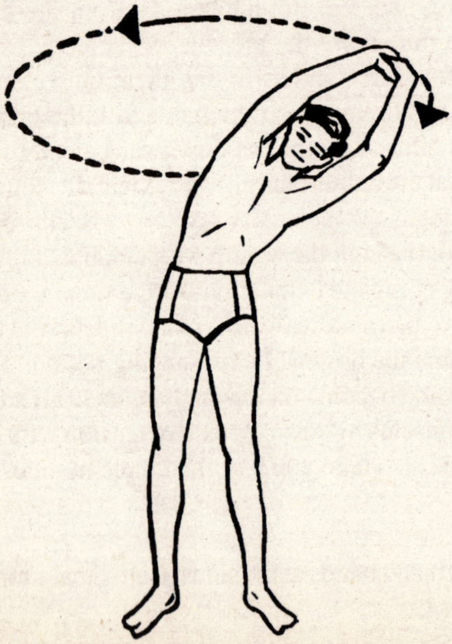

Fig. 6

Cleansing Breaths

After a routine of deep-breathing, or following a set of toning-up exercises, it is a good idea to do several cleansing breaths. These help to expel impurities, strengthen the lower respiratory muscles, and enrich the tone of the voice.

1. The 'Ha' Breath

Standing with feet apart, take a full yoga breath while raising the arms sideways until they meet over your head, palms facing each other. Then without pausing, let the upper part of the body drop forward from the waist, so that the head, torso and arms hang loosely towards the floor. While you did this expel all the air suddenly through the mouth to the sound of 'Ha'. Make sure you drive as much air as possible from the lungs, and relax while you are leaning downward.

Begin to inhale again as you straighten up, sweeping the arms sideways, with palms up, as if you are gathering-in the precious air and *prana*. When the arms are above the head again, drop downward as before, and expel the air noisily again 'Ha'. Repeat this exercise three or four times.

2. The Whistle Breath

Standing with feet apart, take in a full yoga breath through the nose. Purse the lips forward as if you are about to whistle. Now send the air out through the pursed lips in several short bursts. Use the muscles of the abdomen and the diaphragm to drive the air out in this way, until your lungs feel completely empty. Then let the air flow back again by expanding the abdomen, and repeat the exhaling spurts. Do this cleansing exercise three or four times.

PRANAYAMA

Breathing to a particular, pre-determined rhythm, that is with a certain length of time for inhalation, for retention, and for exhalation, can be carried out in various postures: standing, lying flat on your back in the Relaxation Posture, in the Kneeling or one of the cross-legged postures (to be taught in later chapters) or sitting bolt upright in a chair, feet flat on the floor, and hands resting on the knees, palms upward – this latter is sometimes called the Egyptian Posture.

When you have learned to be comfortable in one of the cross legged postures, it is as well to practise most of your breath control and retention exercises (*pranayama*) in that. In such a position you can remain very still, collected, balanced and calm.

The counting during breath control must, of course, be done mentally and kept even and regular throughout. There are several ways of achieving this. You can place two fingers on your pulse at the wrist and use that as a counting guide. If you are able to hear your own heart-beat this will make an easy counting guide for most occasions. Both of these methods are good because they unite the breathing to the rhythm of the blood. If on the other hand you have difficulty in finding your pulse, or hearing your heart-beat, you can use the modern doctor's method of ticking off the seconds by saying mentally, 'thousand-and-one, thousand-and-two, etc.' to represent seconds.

The eventual rhythm to aim for in *pranayama* is the ratio 1:4:2. But you must not attempt this rhythm immediately. Lead up to it gradually.

At first it will be as well not to retain the breath at all. Let your rhythm be 4:4 – counting four while you breathe in, and four while the breath is going out. After practising this for a few days, you can move on to a 4:4:4 rhythm. Count four during inhalation, hold the breath to the count of four, and exhale to four. Later try 6:6:6 counts, and after a few weeks move to another practice rhythm of 4:4:8, and then to 4:8:8.

When you feel that you are really beginning to master your breath control, you can try the advanced 1:4:2 ratio. But before doing that you should have been practising an important breathing exercise called the Bellows.

The Bellows

1. Sitting in one of the cross-legged postures, with the hands resting on the knees, breathe into the upper part of the lungs and out again as quickly as possible. Your chest will be rising and falling like a pair of bellows. Keep the mouth shout and use the nose only. Take a dozen inhalations in this way.
2. In the same posture, breathe deeply into the diaphragm. The bellows are now in the abdomen; press it inwards to exhale, and expand it quickly forwards to inhale. One complete inhalation and exhalation should take only a second, yet you must aim to fill the lower part of the lungs completely at each inhalation. Take a dozen breaths in this manner. Such rapid nasal breathing will of course be noisy for both the shallow and the deep bellows.

Some *Pranayama* Exercises. (Beginning the 1:4:2 ratio)

1. Seated cross-legged, or in one of the other postures described above, exhale completely. Now with two fingers of the right hand on the

pulse in the left wrist, or listening to the heart-beats within, inhale through the nose to three pulse beats, hold the breath to twelve beats, and exhale through the nose to six beats. Do this five times and rest.

2. (*Fig. 7*) While sitting cross-legged, or in one of the appropriate postures, bring the right hand to the face, and place the index finger on the forehead between the eyes; bring the thumb and bent middle finger against the nostrils on each side. Exhale and close the right nostril with the thumb. Draw the air in through the left nostril while you mentally count 'thousand-and-one, thousand-and-two, thousand-and-three'. Fill the lungs in this time. Close the left nostril with the middle finger. Now with both nostrils closed, count up to three seconds in like manner. Open the right nostril, and exhale to the count of three seconds. Immediately breathe in through the nostril to the count of three, press the right thumb onto the right nostril and hold the nose closed while you count to three again. Open the left nostril, and exhale to the count of three. You have now done one round of *pranayamas*. Do *three* more of these and then rest.

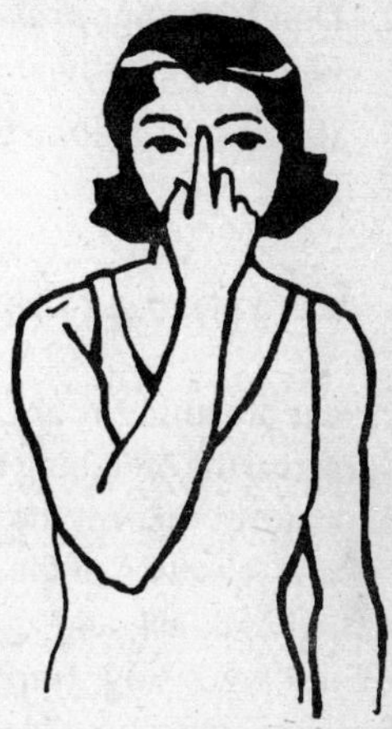

Fig. 7

After some practice, five rounds can be done at one session, but the student should not do more than five at one time.

Warnings

1. Breathing rhythms involving longer breath retention should not be attempted by the student working alone. If attempted at all, it should be under the supervision of a very experienced teacher. Even, in the simple rhythm given here, if the student feels any strain in retaining his breath he should stop the practice, otherwise, he might do himself more harm than good. In the alternate nostril breathing, for example, he could inhale to a comfortable count and, without retaining the breath, exhale to the same count. It is important to enjoy the exercise without any strain.

You may read somewhere that the 'minimum' *pranayama* figures for a Hindu yogi are 12:48:24, but remember this is achieved after years of practice under supervision. It is said that some yogis of the Orient reach the *pranayama* figures in the 1:4:2 rhythm of 36:144:72, and with this their bodies begin to levitate.

2. Don't attempt *pranayama* involving the retention of breath, unless your heart is sound.
3. If you start feeling dizzy during any breathing exercises stop at once for a rest.

HOW TO PRACTISE YOGA BREATHING

Correct breathing is an integral part of the yoga postures, so it is as well to practise the breathing exercises for a week or two before starting to learn the postures (except the Relaxation Posture described in Chapter Two).

Do at least two of the breathing routines described above each morning before breakfast, and again some time during the day or evening.

Start practising simple breath control while in the Relaxation Posture, after you have completely relaxed.

Some While-You-Work Exercises

1. Pause in your activities for three minutes and do one of the three breathing routines given in this chapter, whenever you think of it.
2. Sitting in your car (not while driving), the bus, train, or office do beginners *pranayama*, i.e., the 4:4 or 4:4:4 rhythms using both nostrils, unless you are alone.
3. When walking, sometimes practice what is called 'squared' *pranayama* – that is breathe in as you take four steps, hold it for four steps, exhale while you take four steps, and hold the breath out for the next four steps. Then begin again. This gives the rhythm 4:4:4:4.

Some Benefits

Through continual practice in yoga breathing your normal breathing will automatically improve. This means that the marvelous 'carrier system' of your body – the blood – will be able to work more efficiently. It will convey more oxygen around for tissue repair and renewal; it will carry away the waste matter of cell destruction with a much greater thoroughness. This will lead to a toning-up of the whole body, improvement in general health, more resistance to disease – especially diseases of the chest and lungs.

Deep rhythmic breathing trains the yoga student to control and live by his own individual rhythm, and to harmonise this with the rhythm of the universe. In this way it protects him against harmful and discordant influences both from outside, and from within the human complex. Emotional people become more self-controlled and stable. The spirit is calmed and a deep-seated peace of mind begins to manifest itself within.

Pranayama awakens latent forces dormant in man. Apropos the yoga teaching that it has a direct bearing on length of life, it is interesting to note the relationship between the breathing-rate and the life-span of animals. In general, the slow-breathing animals are not so excitable and live longer than the rapid-breathing ones. A hen for instance breathes about thirty times per minute, a dog about twenty-eight, a monkey about thirty, but the long-living tortoise about three.

The very advanced yogi in *pranayama* breathes only once in four minutes.

A Special Pranayama Exercise

This exercise can be done either sitting, standing or lying on the back. The important thing is to keep the back straight. After clearing the lungs of breath, begin to breathe in slowly through the nostrils sending the prana down the spine while mentally chanting the word *'Om'*, then, without retaining the breath, exhale slowly, imagining the *prana* travelling up the spine while again chanting the word *'Om'*. Repeat the breathing in and breathing out ten times. Do the exercise at least once a day but three times a day if possible. The value of the exercise is that after some practice it brings you a greater control of *prana*, enabling you to send it more easily to any part of the body as required. For example, if you have a pain in the knee joint, or a knuckle joint, you will be able to send an extra supply of *prana* to the joint to heal it. Remember that by feeling right into the spot with the mind you will inevitably bring in the healing *prana*.

CHAPTER FIVE

The Supple Figure of Youth

Our bodies are built on a framework of bone, but if we are not to be fixed immovably to one spot like a tower, the framework must be jointed and hinged at certain points. The structure and location of the joints has been determined by the type of mobility we need for our existence on this earth. They were somehow brought about through the miracle of creative evolution.

The spine, for instance, has to give a certain degree of movement combined with the strength needed as the central column holding the body upright. To achieve this the creative force has placed small bones (the vertebrae) on top of one another, as you would lay bricks. A pad of fibro-cartilage is present between (and attached to) every two vertebrae. This gives the spine necessary flexibility, but more strength than there is in highly movable joints, such as the fingers.

Where circular movement is valuable to man, ball-and-socket joints have been arranged – hemispherical heads fit into cup-shaped sockets, as at the hip and shoulder joints.

Then there are the hinge joints that move like a door in one direction only, such as the knee; and double hinge joints that allow movement in two directions, like a swing door; of this type is the wrist.

In freely movable joints the separate bones that turn, slide or swing on one another are held together by a capsule of ligaments surrounding the joint. The bone surfaces which come into contact are shaped to fit one another accurately, and are covered with a thick glistening pad of smooth cartilage. This acts a buffer between the hard bones, absorbing shock; it also provides a surface on which movement can be made continually without friction and wear to the bones.

In addition there is a synovial membrane strategically placed in the joint to provide a lubricating system. The membrane secretes a thick sticky substance similar to white of egg in appearance and consistency. This is called synovial fluid and serves to keep the joint well nourished and lubricated.

As well as the various ligaments that join the bones at the joints, giving the required strength without detracting too much from the freedom of movement, some joints are provided with extra pads of fibro-cartilage to lessen the risk of dislocation.

Whether our movements will be jerky and awkward or smooth and graceful depends largely on the health and proper functioning of the many joints of the body. To keep them healthy we need to exercise them in the right manner. At the same time they are affected by our general health.

Yet apart from the health of the body in general and of the joints in particular, there is some other factor involved. Why does one person move with the sinuous grace of a panther while another stumps about like a clumsy machine? Why are some sporting people graceful and supple in their actions, while others are just the reverse? Health and physical exercise are not the whole story behind the poetic beauty of motion.

But can we all be as resilient and graceful as the cat and the tiger? Another vital question is this: is it inevitable that our joints should stiffen, that we should lose elasticity, agility, easy movement as we grow older? Time gets the blame for all the rheumaticky creaking and stiffening, but perhaps it is not the main offender after all.

I saw a teenager watching his uncle, who was in his late fifties, doing the Plough posture (touching the ground with his toes behind his head), bending over in Deep Obeisance to put his face between his knees, bending right backward to place his hands on the ground behind, with the whole of his body arched in a posture called the Bridge. The boy was giving gasps of amazement; he was a vigorous lad, keen on sports, but he could not do these things. His uncle was one of the new yogis of the West.

I knew a yoga teacher in his seventies who had the figure and vitality of a man of twenty, and even more suppleness. I have seen both men and women of all ages in yoga classes transformed from awkward, stiff ungainliness, to a smooth flexible grace of form and movement.

While old boxers and athletes often run to weight or to seed, and old soldiers, though rugged, are usually rigid, Hatha yogis and yoginis (women yogis), full of years, retain their slimness and elasticity to the end of life. Why is this?

The main reason lies in that vital integration at which yoga aims – the marriage of mind and body. The yogi not only exercises his joints, he mentally *becomes* his joints as he exercises; his centre of consciousness moves from its usual seat in the brain right into the joints. This creates in time an effortless, fluid coordination of mind and matter. Further, the yoga training leads to more flexibility and resilience of mind, and this in turn is reflected in the body.

The set of yoga exercises given below has been selected to keep all the important hinges of the body well oiled, healthy and pliant. That's one of their functions. The other is to prepare the body for the more advanced work – the yoga postures.

Here are four points to bear in mind concerning the exercises.

1. Do them often.
2. Keep your face relaxed, and smile sometimes, while you are doing them.
3. Keep the mind concentrated on the parts being exercised.
4. Never force muscles and joints too far. Apply gentle pressure only, being guided by your inner judgement about the amount of force to use. It takes only one second to strain a muscle or joint, but many weeks to get them back to normal again.

Neck Routine

Stand with feet apart, or sit in a chair, or sit in a cross-legged posture. Breathe naturally throughout – in fact, don't think about your breathing.

(*a*) Bend the neck as far forward as possible, then as far backward as possible. Four times in each direction.

(*b*) Bend the neck as far sideways as possible. Four times to each side.

(*c*) Turn the head as if to look over the right shoulder. Pause for a moment in that position and mentally observe the pressures in the neck. Turn it as far as possible to the left, and do the same. Do four turns in each direction.

(*d*) Lift the chin as high as possible, until you feel a pleasant stretch in the skin and muscles. Let go, and drop the head loosely onto your chest, relaxing the whole of your face and skull. Do this four times.

(*e*) Swing the head in a circular motion – clockwise and then anti-clockwise – four times in each direction. Make the circle as large as you can, and move the head slowly until the head has become supple, then more quickly. Observe sensations.

At the end gently slap the face and neck all over with both hands, relaxing the tissues.

Routine for a Healthy, Supple Spine

Stand with the feet apart. Breathe naturally, and concentrate attention on the spine and back muscles.

(a) (Fig. 8) Bring both shoulders forward, downward, then backward and upward, in a full, slow circular motion. Do six circles this way, closely observing the feelings in the working muscles and spinal column.

Do six circles in the reverse direction - that is, with the shoulders going forward and upward, then backward and downward. Bend the spine as much as required, and hold the consciousness in the area concerned.

(b) (Fig. 9) Now circle the shoulders alternately, one following the other, with a motion similar to that used in swimming the Crawl. Rotate each slowly upward, forward, downward and backward. Keep the whole body loose, and wriggle the trunk with a snake-like flexibility. After doing six circles with each shoulder, reverse the direction and complete six more circles with each shoulder, in the new direction.

Think of nothing whatever but the pleasant feelings you are creating within your body.

(c) Put your hands on your hips and bend from the waist, forward and then backward as far as possible – four times in each direction. Pause for a moment. Bend over to the right and then over to the left from the waist, feeling the side muscles stretching pleasantly. Do four to the right and four to the left. Pause. Circle from the waist clockwise in large slow circles four times, then immediately change direction and circle anti-clockwise

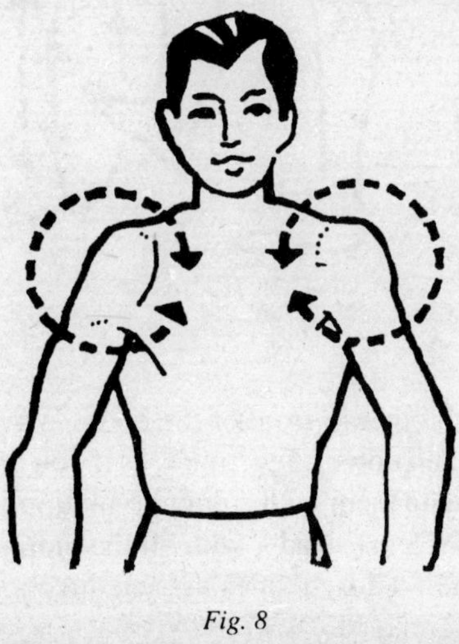

Fig. 8

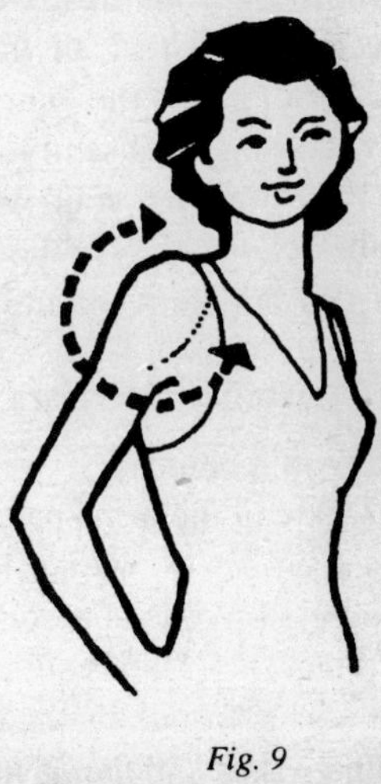

Fig. 9

four times. Keep the lower part of the body from the hips down as steady as possible. Hold the mind on the lower part of the spine and waistline.

Leg Flexibility Exercises

(a) Standing, put the weight on the left leg, and hold onto something (such as a piece of furniture) with your left hand. Swing the right leg, from the hips, forward and backward like a pendulum, as far as you can. Swing it six times or more in each direction. Turn around. Transfer the weight to the right leg, hold the support with your right hand, and swing the left leg in the same manner. The swinging leg should feel loose and easy; the mind should be centred in the hips.

(b) Put the weight on the left leg again, and lift the right leg by bending the knee sharply, about half a dozen times. Transfer the weight and bend the left knee in the same way. In this exercise you must bend each knee as rapidly and as far as possible, but there's no need to lift the knees high. Fasten your attention inside the joints of the knees.

(c) (Fig. 10) Stand on the left leg again, and hold the right leg out in front of you about six inches from the floor. Rotate the right foot from the ankle, clockwise and anti-clockwise – about six times in each direction. Then raise and lower the foot, using the ankle as a hinge, a few times. Next shake the whole leg from the hip to the toes; shake until you feel all the tensions going out of it, and the joints and muscles becoming pleasantly loose and free. Now transfer your weight onto the right leg and give your left the same pleasant, rejuvenating treatment.

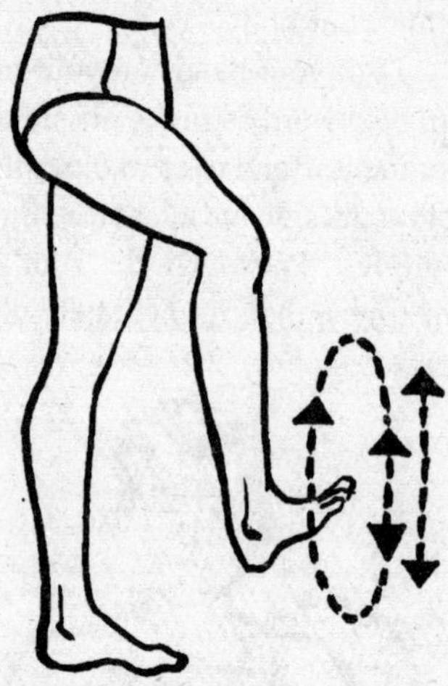

Fig. 10

Arm Flexibility Exercises

Stand with feet apart.

(a) Extend the arms parallel to each other in front of the body. Wave the hands, from the wrists, loosely up and down a few times, as if you are waving goodbye to someone. Then rotate them with a circular motion in both directions. Hands should be loose, arms steady, with all the motion at the wrists. Rotate the hands about half a dozen times in each direction until the wrists and hands feel free and relaxed.

(b) Swing both arms in a circular motion like a windmill, using the ball-and-socket joints of the shoulders as pivots. Let the arms go very relaxed, and do about six circles in each direction.

Now concentrating attention on the elbows, bend the arms sharply, bringing the hands up to touch the shoulders. Keep muscles loose throughout. Do first with separate arms, and then with both together – about six times each.

(c) Raise both arms in front of you and shake them thoroughly so that you feel all the muscles vibrating from shoulders to fingers. At the same time move them freely at the shoulders, elbows and wrists – they should be waving and undulating like two snakes.

The Deep Obeisance Posture *(Fig. 11)*
This is also called the Stork Posture. Its Sanskrit name is *Padahastasana.*

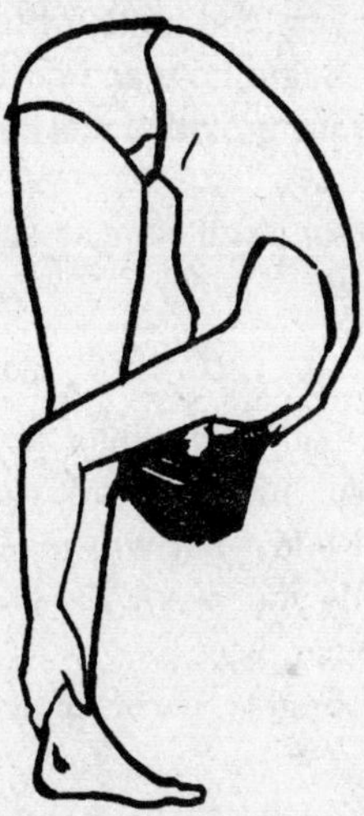

Fig. 11

Phase 1
Stand with the feet together. Raise your arms straight above your head with the palms facing forward. Breathe in.

Phase 2
Breathing out, and drawing the stomach in, bend smoothly forward from the waist and place the palms flat on the ground as near as possible to the toes. Pause a moment, then take hold of your ankles, placing the forearms along the legs, and gently pull until your face touches your knees. Hold the posture while you take three full abdominal breaths.

At first you may not even be able to touch the floor, let along bring the head to the knees. Never mind; don't strain to achieve the position; flexibility will come with practice. Just push the hands as close as you can to the floor, and remaining there, relaxing, take your three full breaths.

Phase 3
Stand up, inhaling deeply as you do so. Bring your arms to their starting position above the head, then let them fall to your sides as you exhale.

Remember, this is not just a gymnastic feat; go down slowly without any jerkiness; keep the mind fully absorbed with the breathing and the muscular pressures of the body.

More important than the feat of reaching your knees with your nose are the great benefits of trying to do so.

You may at first feel dizzy, if so, stop for a rest and proceed slowly. Persist in practice – with moderation – and the dizziness will soon be a thing of the past.

Some Results

The Deep Obeisance makes stiff spines pliable. It stimulates internal organs – stomach, liver, kidneys, intestines – and helps keep them functioning well. It enlivens circulation in the upper parts of the body with great benefit to the brain and nerves.

How to Practise the Exercises

You can run through all the flexibility exercises of this chapter including the Deep Obeisance in eight minutes. That's not much time to give in return for the supple figure of youth – maintained to the very end of your life.

Don't wait until you have finished the book. Begin now and do the whole of this loosening-up set once a day, at any time provided it is three hours after a meal.

Some of these exercises are used to limber-up for a full yoga session, while others are useful for finishing-off the session.

Punctuate your day with these

There are some valuable little flexibility exercises that you can intersperse throughout your ordinary daily activities. They will not only work wonders towards healthy joints and a pliant graceful body, but will relieve mental tension, and create a better attitude towards your work. Do them while you are sitting in the office, the bus, or in other places.

1. Lift and lower the toes of each foot as far as possible. Do separately, then together – as many times as you can.
2. Shake the hands and arms freely – one at a time, then both together. Play imaginary five-finger exercises with the fingers. Open and shut the hands several times quickly to loosen the fingers.
3. Sag the jaw and wag the chin sideways, to right and left, rapidly several times.
4. Poke the tongue out and stretch it forwards as far as it will go several times.
5. Do some of the neck exercises described in this chapter.

CHAPTER SIX

Build Your Body as You Want It

Many physical culture systems have proved that big bulging muscles can be created out of puny ones. But there are risks in this. One danger is that you may become 'muscle-bound' – restricted in movement within your prison of ponderous muscles. Another is that you many finish up as a slave to your over-developed muscular system – working hard to maintain it, so that it will not turn to flabby fat. But if you are interested in yoga, you will not be interested in building these big showy muscles. What should you aim at then? Stand in front of a long mirror – minus your clothes – and take a close critical look at that physical vehicle of yours. No matter how excellent it is, it will not be perfect. There will be flabby places, bulges where there should be flatness, flatness where there should be bulges.

Your objective is to remove the surplus fat, to make flabby flesh attractively firm, to create a smooth, adequately-developed muscular system so that your body has neat symmetry, as well as grace. You want to keep all your muscles well toned-up, infused with the fundamental life force – the *prana* – so that they glow with health and strength.

In short, your aim is to turn your physical vessel into a thing of beauty. Beauty is something that you *can* create for yourself, but you must remember that it is never entirely physical. Even in a very physical thing, such as an oil painting or a marble statue, if it has true beauty, there is some spiritual quality imparted by the artist. This non-physical quality must enter still more into the creation of a beautiful physical body. It derives really from the inner essence of yoga, from the union of all the parts of a human being – physical, mental and spiritual.

I have seen many examples of how this true beauty of body can be created by the artist within, when he makes use of the potent yoga technique.

I recall particularly a very stout, stiff-bodied woman in her early forties who came along to a yoga class. She had used a great variety of diets in a valiant but losing battle against encroaching avoirdupois. The yoga class was, I believe, a kind of last resort for her.

I watched her struggle heroically with the exercises and postures. For the first weeks there seemed to be no tangible results at all, but the woman had grit; she kept at it, and eventually the visible change began. Six months after she started she was more than four stone lighter, which was the correct weight for her height. At the end of a year you would not have known her for the same woman. She was supple of figure, and was aglow with vitality. Eventually she became one of the class's leading demonstrators on yoga postures. Her figure and her life had both changed completely.

I have seen scrawny men put on weight through doing the same exercises and postures. Yoga brings you to your *right* weight, increasing it where necessary – putting on firm rounded muscles; reducing it if you are overweight – pricking the 'spare tyres', deflating middle-age spread, burning up adipose tissue. And all this without any special diet, other than the sensible moderate eating recommended by yoga.

These apparent miracles of change depend not only on the muscle-toning exercises given in this chapter, but on the whole yoga system. *Pranayama,* for example, plays a dominant part in the adjustment of weight.

But we *do* have a duty – a pleasant one – towards our muscular apparatus. Let us have a look at what muscles are and how they work. In a medium-sized muscle there are ten million cells with each cell made up of 400 little fibres. This means 4,000 million fibres – or working parts – in the muscle. Amongst these bundles of fibres run nerves and blood vessels.

The 639 muscles of the body are attached at each end to bone – or, more rarely, to skin. They are the body levers, ropes and pulleys, with the main function of moving parts of the bony framework through one or more of its hundred joints.

They make their pull on the bones by contracting or shortening, but the power behind the pull, the force that sets things in motion, comes from outside the muscles by way of the nerves.

When, for instance, your mind desires to stretch the hand in a certain direction and pick up a cup, a force – an electrical impulse – goes along the nerves into the millions of cells of the appropriate muscles. Blood brings water, protein, hormones, enzymes, sugar for fuel and oxygen –

ready for combustion. Bang! With perfect precision the ten million cells in each muscle explode. (Scientists have a machine that will pick up the explosive sound of a contracting muscle.)

This combustion creates the kind of activity that makes the muscles contract, thereby giving the degree of force to carry out the required action. Blood carries away the waste products of the explosion. This is helped by the contracting muscles squeezing down on the blood vessels, and pushing the blood, laden with the waste products, along towards the heart. Then as the muscles relax again, pure arterial blood rushes in. In this way muscular exercise aids your circulation, and makes it easier for your heart to do its work properly.

Even a simple action, like picking up a cup of tea, requires the use of several muscles, and each has to receive its electrical impulse from the nerves, and have its little explosion. The forces thus set up must be accurately balanced and related, so that the pulls and resistances are in exact coordination. Otherwise something goes wrong – the hand misses the cup, or knocks it over, or lifts it too suddenly and spills the contents. Movements of the body are really very complex, coordinated operations that demand close subtle integration of forces.

Muscles are the physical parts of us that can most easily be increased in size and strength by mental action. They respond amazingly to the Unconscious Mind. If you do not use a muscle, the Unconscious will quickly decide that the muscle cannot be of value, and let it fade away and atrophy. Think how your leg muscles reduce in size when you are sick and inactive in bed for a few weeks.

If, on the other hand, you regularly exercise a muscle, the Unconscious Mind decides that this particular lever must be of great importance. It is, therefore, not only given the energy to do what you ask, but its size and strength are built up so that it is able to do even harder work than you are demanding. It thrives on work, increasing its potentiality for more, gaining all the time in dimension, health, tone and vigour.

The yoga technique concentrates the intelligence, imagination and will on directing unconscious forces in muscle formation. When you are doing the muscle-toning exercises you visualise the kind of body you want; you picture its slimness, its well-rounded resilient muscles, its firm abdomen and hips. Your will-power helps the mental and nerve forces to burn away the superfluous rolls of fat, to make firm the sagging tissues.

The more clearly and vividly you can picture that human form of health and beauty, which is your goal, the sooner you will achieve it. While you exercise, assist the Unconscious Builder within; speed up his good work by centering your conscious attention inside the muscle; enjoy its activity; increase the flow of vital life force in the cells. Affirm your objectives. Say mentally to yourself: - 'My muscles are growing firm, strong, vital ... my superfluous fat is being burned away ... my figure is becoming slim, lithe, youthful' – or whatever other results you desire. Work and think with conviction, and your aims will surely materialise.

Throughout the following exercises breathe naturally, and try to achieve a rhythm between tension and relaxation in the muscles concerned.

EXERCISES FOR TONING-UP THE MUSCLES AND BEAUTIFYING THE BODY

Leg Work

(1) *(Fig.12)* Stand with feet apart. Bend the knees forward, inward, downward toward each other, bringing them as near together as possible. Straighten up and relax. Repeat this six times.

(2a) *(Fig. 13)* Stand with left foot ahead of right some eighteen inches. Bend both knees forward, pressing the rear knee towards the ground as much as possible. Press it down about six times, feeling the tension in the calf of the rear leg. Change the position of the legs, putting the right forward, and repeat the six downward presses.

(2b) With the legs in the same position, one front of the other as if taking a step, practise 'running on the spot' – that is, without moving the

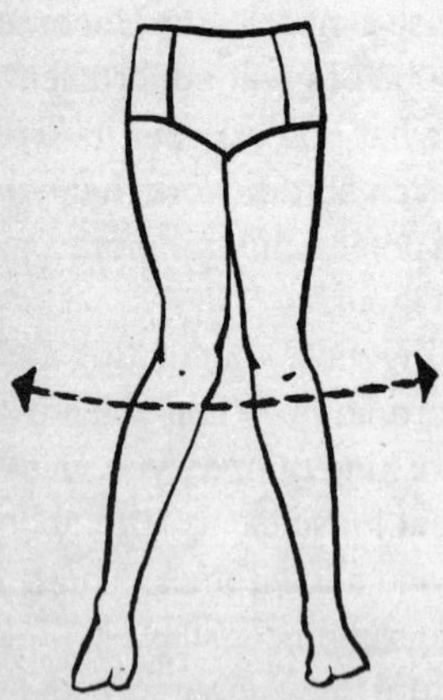

Fig. 12

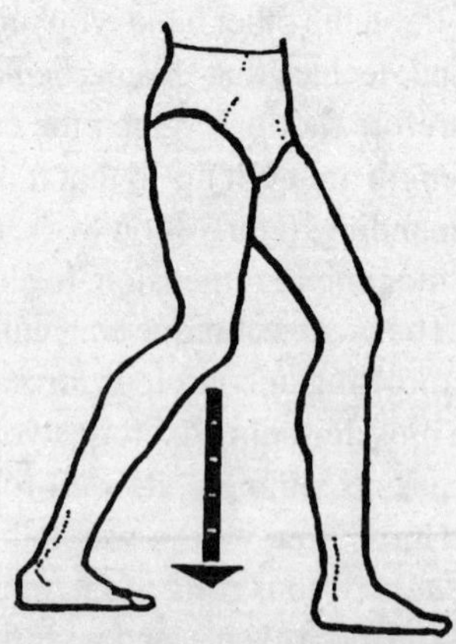

Fig. 13

feet from the floor, work the muscles of the legs alternately as if you are running. Feel every muscle in the legs as you try to propel yourself forward. Exercise with each foot forward in turn.

(3) With heels together rise high on the toes a dozen times.

Remember to keep the whole mental attention on the stresses in the muscles of the legs throughout the above exercises.

Arm Work *(Fig. 14)*

Standing with feet apart and hands at sides, close the fists and bend the arms at the elbows, slowly bringing the fists forward and upward towards the shoulders. Feel the tension in the biceps. When the arms are bent as much as possible at the elbows and wrists, with the closed hands leaning towards the shoulders, slowly turn the hands in a half-circle outward away from the shoulders feeling the pressures in the muscles as you do so. Drop the arms to the sides and shake them gently to relax them. Then repeat. Do this exercise about six times to completely tone-up the arms. Hold the consciousness in the arms throughout.

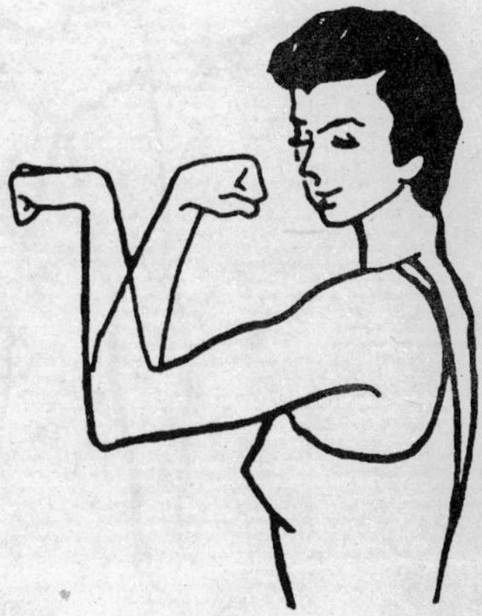

Fig. 14

Back Work

Stand with feet apart. Bend the knees and go down as if you are about to pick up a bar lying on the ground in front of your toes. Grasp the imaginary bar and rise very slowly. It is a heavy bar; you must feel and enjoy the tension in all your back muscles. Keep your mind in these muscles.

When you are standing upright again with your hands at your sides, consciously relax the back muscles. Repeat the bar-lifting movement, with back tensing and relaxing, six times.

Chest Work *(Fig. 15)*

Stand with feet apart and hands at the sides. Raise the arms outward until they are about eighteen inches away from the body. Now bring them in towards the body, tensing the muscles of the chest. When the arms have reached the body, let go the tension, swing the arms together in front of the body, and then take them slowly outward, tensing the chest muscles

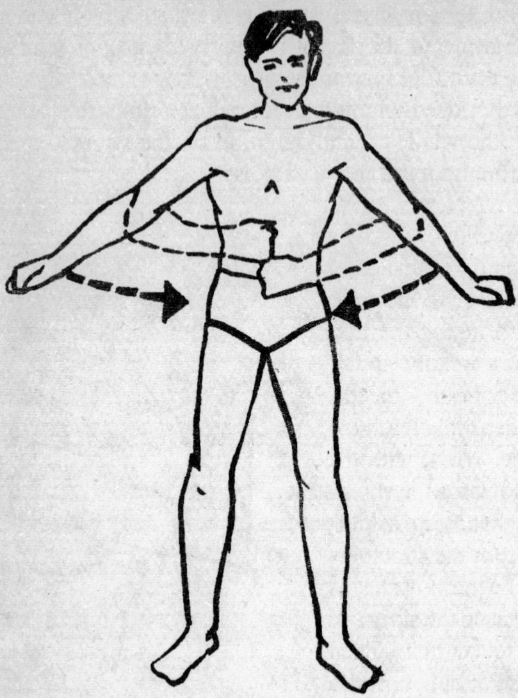

Fig. 15

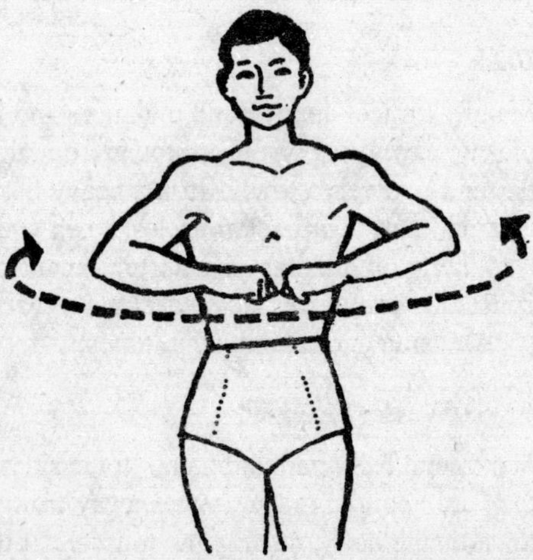

Fig. 16

again as the arms move out to the position about eighteen inches from the sides of the body.

Then let the arms fall to the sides, shake them to relax the chest muscles. Remember, in this exercise the attention must not be in the arms; they should remain relaxed throughout.

You are toning-up the chest muscles and that is where your mind must be directed.

Repeat the exercise twelve times.

Exercises for Abdomen *(Fig. 16)*

(1) Stand with feet apart. Close the hands loosely and raise them to the level of the breast so that they are a few inches apart, and the elbows are pointing sideways. Now put the attention on the muscles at each side of the abdomen, and swing the shoulders to the right and then to the left as far as possible. You should continue to look straight ahead with the head steady, so that only the trunk turns, pivoting on the neck above and the hips below. Feel the pleasant stretching of the abdominal muscles as you swing the shoulders rhythmically from side to side. Do about six turns in each direction.

You will probably find that this exercise releases gas that has collected in the stomach.

(2) Lie down on your back (either on the carpet or on a folded rug). Relax your body and place your hands gently on your abdomen. Breathe out.

As you slowly inhale, raise your legs and bend your knees, bringing them up so that your thighs comes as close as possible to your abdomen. Pause for a moment, filling the lungs completely.

Retaining the breath, straighten your legs so that you are holding them stretched upwards at an angle of about forty-five degrees from the floor. Now lower them as slowly as you can to the floor while you exhale.

With your hands you will feel the keen tension in the working muscles. Use mind and hand-movement to relax the abdomen completely when the feet return to the floor.

Visualise the firm flat abdomen you wish to produce and retain. Make the appropriate mental affirmations. Repeat the exercise from six to a dozen times, depending on your strength, and your needs in the removal of surplus fat.

Combining Exercises with Daily Activities

Any of the exercises can, of course, be done at odd moments if you happen to be alone or with some sympathetic companions. Otherwise there are some valuable things that can be carried out, without anyone knowing it, while you are sitting or standing at work, or while travelling.

Here are four:

(1) Select a muscle of your body to tense, relax, and mentally observe. It is easier at the start to choose a leg or arm muscle for this. Try to tense and relax it. Perhaps at first it will not respond. But just making the attempt has a good effect, and eventually the muscle will come under your conscious control.

(2) When standing – waiting for your bus or for some other reason – practise Leg Work No. 3. Tense and relax all the muscles of the legs as you rise on the toes.

(3) Inhale and hold the breath. Tense all the muscles of the abdomen. Prod them with your fingers. Relax and exhale.

(4) Try simultaneous tensing and relaxing of two separate muscles in different parts of they body. Pairs to exercise together could be, for instance, left forearm and left calf, right forearm and right calf, left hip and right side of chest, and vice versa; you can choose other combinations for yourself. Exercise a pair about six times, and then rest.

It will help to put a hand on a difficult muscle that you are trying to influence. Don't be discouraged if at first you feel no movement at all. Keep practising.

In this way you will gradually bring many muscles of your body under control of the conscious mind in a marvellous manner, gaining greatly in health, vigour, concentration and will-power.

Remember, your body is created, and continually recreated, by mental and psychic forces. To the extent that you can learn to dominate this by your Conscious Will, you can build your body as you want it to be.

CHAPTER SEVEN

Good Balance, Posture and Poise

Balance is a basic factor of existence. There must be a balance of positive and negative charges inside the atom, otherwise matter would disintegrate and the universe cease to exist.

It is essential for life. Both vegetables and animals have a built-in sense of balance. Vegetable life grows towards the light, spreading its foliage in a way that maintains its erect posture, bending with flexibility before the storm, but always returning to its upright equilibrium. Animals have a natural dynamic balance in movement, and a sure static balance in rest. Some birds, for instance, sleep standing on one leg, others resting on the swaying branch of a tree.

Man has a special problem of balance. He is the only vertebrate who has to maintain equilibrium for long periods in a vertical position. Unfortunately he rarely achieves a posture of perfect balance either in movement or rest. His incorrect balance means ungainly appearance, constant nervous strain, derangement of internal organs and bad health.

More than once I have seen bad posture cause spinal curvature, humped back, hollow chest, resulting after some years in weak lungs, asthma, strained heart and premature death. Prolapses, protruding stomachs, can be prevented by giving attention to the balance of forces working on the body. Many diseases are due to the imbalance of subtle positive and negative currents that can be kept in equilibrium through yoga exercises.

Of course, Nature has endowed man with a sense of balance; otherwise he could not exist. Perhaps if his way of life had remained close to nature this sense would have been as excellent to his purpose as that of other animals is to theirs. But he has moved a long way from natural living, and his sense of balance now needs re-educating and developing – to fortify him, and bring better health and euphoria, amid the stresses of busy urban life.

Yoga aims to do this. Here again it begins, but does not end, with the body. Good balance and posture in the physique engenders a corresponding balance in mind and personality. Yoga works on all aspects of the person. When body, mind and emotions are maintained in good balance – whether in motion or rest – we say that the person has that rare quality known as 'poise'.

While all yoga exercises help towards this end, there are several postures specially designed to educate the sense of balance. Apart from developing the power to adjust the interacting forces that affect the body, yoga postures will encourage you to observe these forces.

Are you walking or standing, for example, with your shoulders slouched forward instead of well back? Are you sitting in that tense cross-kneed position that most people adopt, instead of with both feet on the floor? Do you rely entirely on your back muscles when picking up a heavy weight instead of assisting the back muscles by bending the knees? Are all your movements in sport, games and work carried out with dynamic balance? If not, they will be harmful to the body. Are you putting too much strain on your brain, your nerves, your eyes, your heart? Watch always to maintain a healthy balance of effort in your activities.

Practise regularly the following exercises and postures to acquire an equilibrium of the forces to which you are subjected.

The Tree Posture *(Fig. 17)*

Phase 1

Stand erect with shoulders back and arms to the sides. Transfer all your weight onto your left foot, and pause to get your balance; then lift the right foot and place it on the left thigh with the sole against the inner part of the thigh as high above the knee as you can manage. Place the palms of the, hands together and hold them in front of the chest in a gesture of prayer. Stay in this position for a few seconds breathing naturally, and mentally picturing yourself, as if from outside, standing there perfectly balanced.

Phase 2 (Fig. 18)

While you remain standing on the left leg, take hold of the right foot and bring it up to rest on the front of the left thigh with the heel as near as possible to the groin. Now take the arms above the head with palms together like a pointed arch. Remain for a few seconds in that position as you did in Phase 1.

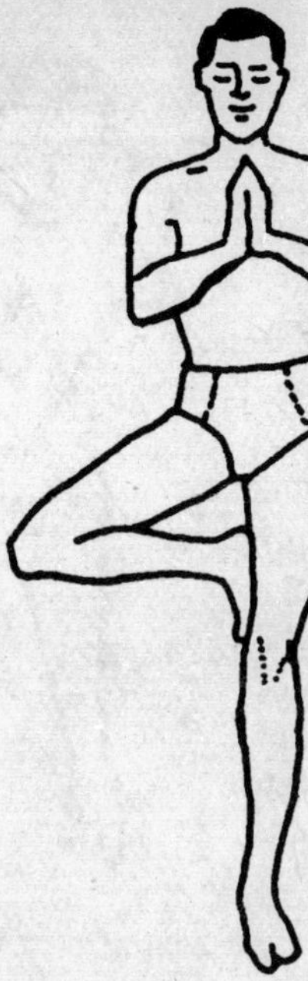

Fig. 17

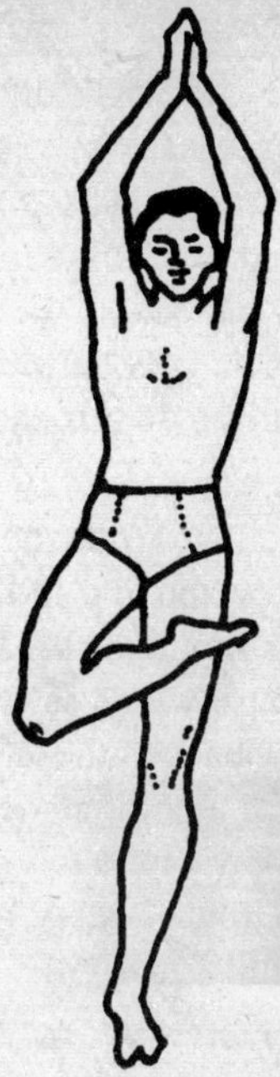

Fig. 18

Phase 3

Still with weight on the left leg, drop the right foot from the front of the thigh, take it in the right hand and hold it behind you. Keep the left hand raised above your head in line with the body, palm facing forward. Hold for a few seconds as in other phases. Finally bring the right foot down and arms to the sides. Relax for a moment, and repeat the three phases of the Tree with the left leg raised.

Points to Note

At the beginning, stand near to something you can hold on to should you start to lose balance. With practice, increase the length of time you stand in each phase. Eventually, as your sense of balance improves, try shutting your eyes as you stand on one leg. In doing this you will need to concentrate very hard on mentally picturing yourself steadily in the erect position.

In this, as in all postures, let movements be smooth and slow, and do not be disheartened by lack of success. It will be easier each time you try because you are educating a natural instinct. Breathe naturally throughout all phases of the posture.

The Corkscrew Posture *(Fig. 19)*

Also called The Eagle, or *Garudasana* in Sanskrit.

Phase 1

Stand erect. Bend the left knee. Cross the right knee over it, and wind the leg around so that the right foot is locked behind the left calf. Bend forward a little and hold your balance steadily in that position. When you can do this easily, pass on to Phase 2.

Phase 2

Rest the left elbow on the right thigh and place the other elbow above it in the crook of the left arm. The hands should be held together lightly, and the wrists bent inwards as shown in figure. Rest the chin on the back of the left (upper) hand, and focus the eyes on a point somewhere beyond the tip of the nose. Hold for a few seconds – or longer with practice. Unwind, relax, and repeat with the opposite legs and arms.

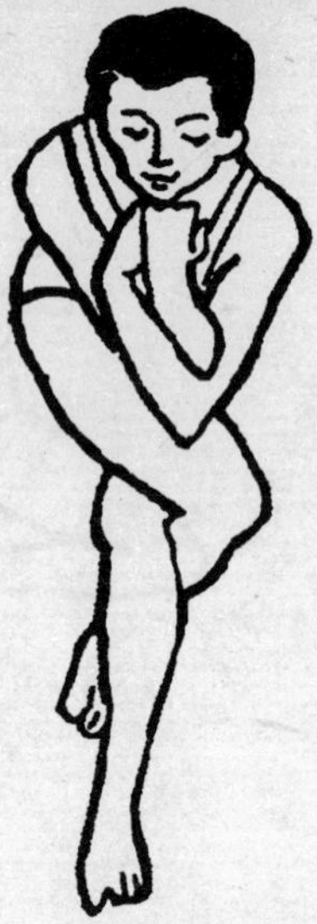

Fig. 19

Points to remember

1. Breathe naturally throughout the posture.
2. Until you have learned to keep your balance in Phase 1, stand near to something that you can hold on to if it becomes necessary.
3. As well as educating your sense of balance, and bringing your body further under command of your will, this posture strengthens legs, knees and ankles.

ABDOMINAL CONTRACTIONS

These, amongst the most important of all yoga exercise, are designed to counteract the bad posture which, with advancing years, cause prolapse of the stomach. At the same time they help to keep digestion working well and prevent constipation.

Uddiyana

Phase 1

Stand with feet about eighteen inches apart, take a full yoga breath, exhale and lean forward, bending the knees a little and placing the hands on the thighs. Suck the stomach in as far as possible towards the spine, creating a deep hollow under the ribs. Hold for a few seconds; then relax, straighten up, and inhale a full deep breath.

You may not at first be able to move your stomach more than an inch or two, but after a few weeks you will create the deep cavity without difficulty.

Phase 2

Instead of retaining the abdomen steadily in a deep hollow, draw it in and let it go again several times. In other words, alternately contract and relax the abdominal muscles. The in-and-out movement of the abdomen may be a quick flapping action, or a slower rolling motion – both are equally effective. Start with half a dozen contractions at a time, and increase it to ten. There is no advantage in exceeding ten contractions in a round, on one exhalation.

At first do two rounds of Phase 1, followed by two rounds of Phase 2 (with six to ten contractions in each). Later the number of rounds can be increased to half a dozen or more of each phase, if your purpose is to deflate 'spare tyres' or combat constipation.

Nauli *(Fig. 20)*

This is an advanced form of abdominal contraction that most people will find difficult, and some will never master. But the benefits are such that it is well worth attempting; even if you do not succeed, you will have gained benefit from the regular concentrated effort of trying.

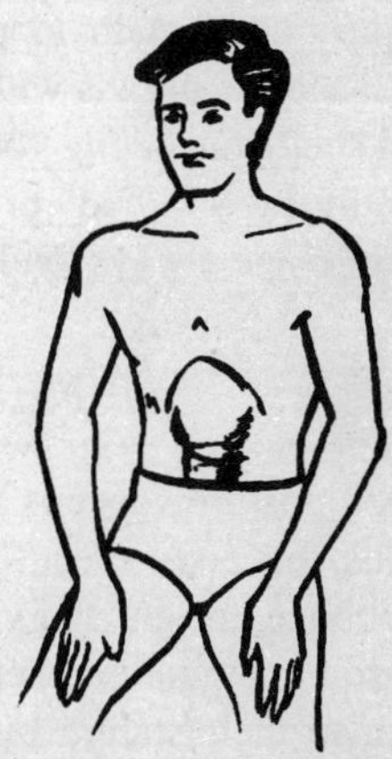

Fig. 20

Execution

The position and breathing are the same as for Uddiyana. When you have made the stomach into a cavity, concentrate the mind on the abdominal recti muscles in the pit of the stomach, just above the pubic bone. Try to contract these to form a hard column, right up the centre of the abdomen.

Follow this immediately by contracting the muscles to the right side, then in the centre again, and then to the left side. In each position a hard muscular column is formed.

When these contractions are performed quickly, one following the other, a continuous churning movement is produced, which to an observer looks like one action, with the column rolling from side to side, instead of a series of three actions.

The posture requires that you bring under control certain muscles that do not normally respond to conscious volition. It will help to close your eyes and picture what you are trying to do. Mentally make a *forward* and *downward* movement in the pit of the stomach; see the column of separated muscle in your mind's eye; one day you will find it there in reality.

Points and Warnings

1. Uddiyana should sometimes be practised in the sitting cross-legged position – the Easy, Perfect, or the Lotus – instead of standing.
2. Never do these abdominal contractions for at least three hours after a meal. The best time to do them are first thing in the morning before breakfast, or before other meals.
3. Women should not do then during menstruation or pregnancy.

Age-delaying Benefit

Geriatrics, the study of senility, is confirming what yoga has long known, that constipation is one of the main causes of ageing in the human being. As we get older the eliminative system becomes sluggish; waste matter, impurities, remain to poison the system. But abdominal contractions massage the organs within, stimulate them to healthy eliminative action, and keep you *feeling* youthful, whatever your age. They keep you *looking* youthful too in body profile – counteracting the barrel-like stomach that middle-age always tends to bring.

SPINE-STRETCHING EXERCISE

Good posture depends a great deal on that important central column that holds the body erect. The following exercises will not only keep the backbone upright and youthful but, if practised enough, can even make a person grow taller. Men in their middle-age have added as much as an inch to their stature by doing the stretching exercise daily for several months.

Execution

Phase 1

Stand with feet together, hands at sides, Without moving the heels from the ground try to stretch the body upward as if, with the top of your head, you would touch an imaginary bar some inches above you. This will tend to straighten out the curves in the spine and stretch the neck. Picture yourself growing taller.

Relax, and then press the body downwards. Do not, of course, bend for this, but – as if there is a great weight on your head – imagine yourself being pressed shorter and shorter.

Repeat the stretching and compressing several times, breathing naturally throughout.

Phase 2

With the arms straight above the head stretch upward trying to reach an imaginary bar with your finger-tips. Stretch one arm, then the other, the together.

Drop the arms and relax. Then press downwards as in Phase 1.

Related Mental Exercise

Stretch the arms above the head with the palms turned forwards; look upwards. This is the gesture of beseeching. Hold it for a while, breathing easily and thinking of Peace.

If you have a worry or problem, stretch as high as possible while you imagine that you are putting your problem up there, above your finger-tips, and leaving it there to be solved by a Power greater and higher than your ordinary, everyday Ego. Bring your arms down and relax, knowing that you have nothing more to worry about. Do this whenever you feel worried or have a problem too great for your thinking mind. You will be surprised at the positive results.

PRACTICE WHILE YOU WORK AND PLAY

Apart from the set exercises and postures given in this chapter, which should be practised at least three times a week, there are several valuable things that can be done during your ordinary activities.

1. Whenever you find yourself sitting with knees crossed, uncross them and sit relaxed with both feet on the floor.
2. From time to time when you are standing or walking, turn the palms of the hands forwards. This will throw the elbows and shoulders back, straighten the spine and keep the head erect. When you turn the palms inwards again towards the legs, keep the arms and shoulders back.
3. Sometimes when you are standing, practise the preliminary position of the Tree – that is, put all your weight on one foot, placing the other foot lightly on top of it, with the knee and toes turned outward. Balance yourself carefully with your eyes open, then close them and see how long you can remain steady. This is excellent practice in balance.

CHAPTER EIGHT

Sense-Control and Sitting Postures

Our troubles, conflicts and sorrows all arise from three sources – from nature, from other people and from within ourselves.

As our understanding deepens, we begin to realise that the inner field of struggle is the important one and that the key to all problems really lies within ourselves. If a man could resolve his inner conflicts, and reach a true unity there, none of the storms from outside would affect him.

Of course, such a man may still battle with the hostilities of Nature, trying to offset her droughts, to guard against her floods, to outwit her microbes. He may still need to wrestle with the lower forces – the ignorance and perversities of mankind. Life would therefore continue to be a struggle.

But the struggle would not really affect him; he would play the drama of life as an actor plays on the stage – knowing its transitory, unreal nature. He would have acquired the invisible armour of protection that yoga calls non-attachment.

Yoga training leads inevitably towards this goal, but we must begin early to practise deliberate sense-control. This is the ability to withdraw attention from what is stimulating any of the five senses – to 'switch-off' the sensory apparatus that connects us with the world outside.

Sound waves in the air may still be hammering against the ear drums, playing on the auditory nerves; sights may be passing before the eyes stimulating the optic nerves, but we will not be aware of them; they will not reach the 'inner senses.'

Some people have learned by experience to concentrate on mental problems in the midst of a noisy crowd. But the majority are too much the victims of their environment; they spend all their time reacting to the stimuli around them – to people, the weather, the newspapers, the television, the clock, the telephone. Their thinking and their moods change accordingly. Life is all outward looking, and there is no inner point of quietness.

How very much the men and women of today need to learn the wonderful art of withdrawal which the sages of Sanskrit writings called *pratyahara.*

Through yoga training deep levels of sense-control can be achieved. The yogi withdraws within his tower of silence, and the noisy bazaar around him becomes as peaceful as a desert place. Scientists have used modern instruments, such as the electroencephalograph, to test objectively the reactions of yoga students in the initial levels of sense-control. Shock effects were shown to be greatly reduced, the 'pain threshold' was raised to a level where unpleasant stimuli caused no observable, or greatly diminished, reactions. Electrical activity was withdrawn completely from the muscular nerves.

But the good effects are really immeasurable. *Pratyahara* calms the nervous system and conserves the energy of the body.

The expenditure of energy by a normal person during eight hours of waking rest is about 750 calories. During the same period of sleep it is about 600 calories. One of the effects of yoga relaxation and *pratyahara* is to reduce the energy expenditure in waking rest to a level even below the figure for sleep. In this way it revitalises and rejuvenates the body so that less sleep is necessary, and advanced yogis scarcely need to sleep at all.

Apart from its value on the deeper levels, *Pratyahara* can have surprising effects in the affairs of daily life.

Once when my wife and I were motoring in a foreign country, we found ourselves detained by the police. It was a totalitarian country; recent political events had brought suspicion on all foreigners, and we had been travelling, inadvertently, through a forbidden area.

We understood enough of the language to appreciate that we were being held on suspicion of spying. Our first urge was, of course, the normal one of protesting, arguing, pleading our innocence. Instead we practised *pratyahara*; we withdrew from the scene of hostility and excitability around us, and sat as calm and remote as statues. This was not, of course, just 'an act'; our long yoga training had taught us to make the inward adjustment, and we were really withdrawn and non-attached.

Soon the atmosphere began to change; the hostile vibrations seemed to be neutralised; a quietness stole over the place. In less than half an hour our passports were returned to us. There was no word spoken – just a half-smile and a gesture to tell us we could be on our way.

Such experiences suggest that when the surface currents are calmed, a deeper Power can go to work for you – not only within, but around you as well.

The power of withdrawal is not achieved through one yoga technique alone. Many work towards it – relaxation, breath-control and postures *(asanas).*

It can and should be practised in the Relaxation Pose, but on the whole the best positions in which to develop sense-control are the various yoga cross-legged postures. At first these may not seem much use for this, or for any other purpose. They will be painful, unless you are very young, because the effects of advancing years usually show themselves first in the joints. The poisons and evil humours must be driven out of the hips and knees and ankles with will-power and practice before you can sit with serenity in the Lotus or the Perfect Postures.

But the pain is, itself, a valuable part of the yoga training and discipline. Its benefits are reaped on all planes – physical, mental and spiritual. Yet never force too much; do not take your movements far beyond the edge of the pain; be content to progress slowly in loosening your joints. It does not matter if you take months – even years – to develop the Lotus Seat. The pain endured is small compared with the benefits gained from the work. As you overcome the stubborn tyranny of your joints, and can sit with ease in some of the traditional cross-legged *asanas,* you will feel something of their mysterious joy and power. They will enable you to concentrate the currents of the body, shut the doors against the outer senses and withdraw into the temple of the undistracted mind.

SITTING EXERCISES AND POSES

The sitting exercises given here help to relax and loosen the joints ready for the cross-legged postures. In the Easy Pose, and other cross-legged postures, the back and neck should be erect in one straight line; the hands may rest on the knees in a relaxed manner, or alternatively they may be placed between the thighs near the body, with the back of the right hand in the palm of the left, and the palms upward.

Head-to-Knee Stretching

Exercise 1

Sit on a flat firm surface with right leg stretched forward and the left bent so that its ankle comes under the right thigh just above the knee. The body is held erect, and the arms loosely at the sides. Take a deep yoga breath. Exhale as you bend slowly forward trying to bring the forehead down to the right knee. At the same time slide the hands forward to clasp the right ankle or foot. Pause there a moment. Inhale as you sit upright again, then repeat the forward movement once.

Change legs so that the left is stretched forward, resting on the right ankle, and do the same forward-stretching exercise twice to that side.

Exercise 2 (Fig. 21)

Instead of putting the ankle of one leg under the thigh of the other, place it so that the sole of the foot is pressed against the inside of the thigh. Then do the forward stretching exactly as in Exercise 1. With the hands holding the forward ankle pull gently to bring the face as close as possible to the knee, but be careful not to strain.

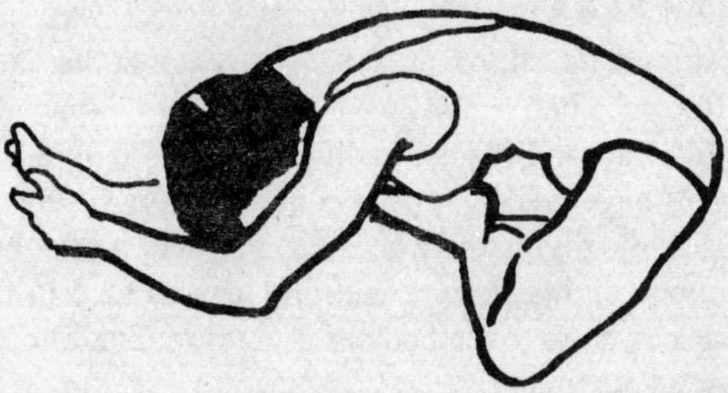

Fig. 21

Exercise 3

When your joints have become sufficiently supple, try the forward stretching with the foot placed, not *below* or *against,* but *on* the thigh of the other leg. The sole of the foot resting on the thigh should be turned upward as much as possible.

Exercise 4 (Fig. 22)

(This is called the Forward-Stretching Posture, *Paschimotanasana* in Sanskrit.)

Sit with both legs stretched in front, feet together, spine and head erect. Inhale. While exhaling and contracting the stomach, bend forward slowly.

Take hold of the ankles or feet and pull gently so that the face comes down as near as possible to the knees. Pause a moment, then inhale as you sit upright.

Perhaps you won't get far down, but don't worry, with practice and gentle persuasion, you will soon be burying your face between your knees, and enjoying it.

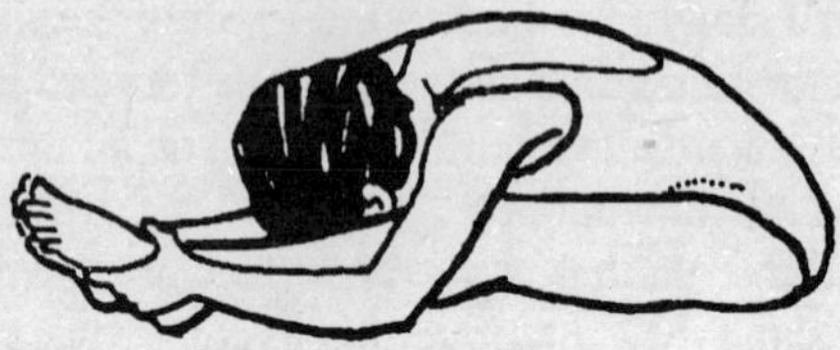

Fig. 22

When you have reached that stage, practise the variation of remaining in the forward bent position while you take three or four deep yoga breaths. This full forward-stretching exercise should be done three or four times at a session.

Exercises in the Easy Posture

The Easy Posture is the simple cross-legged seat that our early ancestors must have often used before the invention of chairs. Many Orientals still prefer to sit this way, and it's the traditional seat of tailors at work. Even in recent years I have seen European country tailors sitting cross-legged on a table-top while plying their needles. You will no doubt be familiar with this common sitting posture with the legs crossed in front and the feet drawn back as close to the body as is comfortable. The knees should be kept as low as possible.

Exercise 1

Sit in the Easy Pose. Clasp the knees with the hands. Rotate the trunk on the buttocks in a clockwise direction making circles as large as possible. As you go forward push the stomach out, and as you go backward draw the stomach in, making it hollow. When you have completed half a dozen wide circles, change direction and rotate anti-clockwise for as many circles. Breathe naturally throughout. Keep the mind on the abdomen.

As well as loosening the hip joints, this exercise fans the digestive fires, and keeps the bowels active.

Exercise 2

After completing the above exercise, remain in the Easy Pose, take a deep breath, and as you exhale, lean over to touch the right knee with the forehead, sliding hands under knees. Return to the upright position inhaling.

Then exhaling again bring the forehead down to touch the left knee. Do this several times to each side. Be content to go as close to the knee as you can manage without strain. In this exercise concentrate the mind on relaxing the upper part of the body.

Exercise 3 (Fig. 23)

Upon completion of Exercise 2, take a full yoga breath; exhale and at the same time lean forward as far as you can, bringing the hands under the knees and trying to touch the floor with the forehead. Pause a moment, and then sit up inhaling. Repeat two or three times.

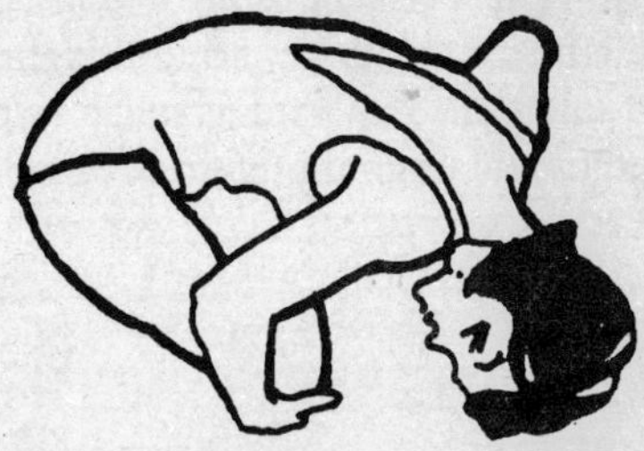

Fig. 23

Posture of Reintegration

After bending forward as in Exercise 3, *remain* in the forward position with the head on, or near, the floor, and breathe deeply for several seconds. Consciously relax any tensions in the face.

Variation. Instead of bringing the hands forwards under the knees, stretch them behind the back and grasp the left wrist with the right hand.

The Perfect Posture, or the Pose of an Adept *(Fig. 24)*

Sitting on your rug with your legs stretched in front of you, fold in the left leg with the left foot as near to the body as possible. Push the heel as far into the groin as you can. Then fold the right leg and insert the edge of the right foot lightly between the thigh and calf of the left leg. The upper heel

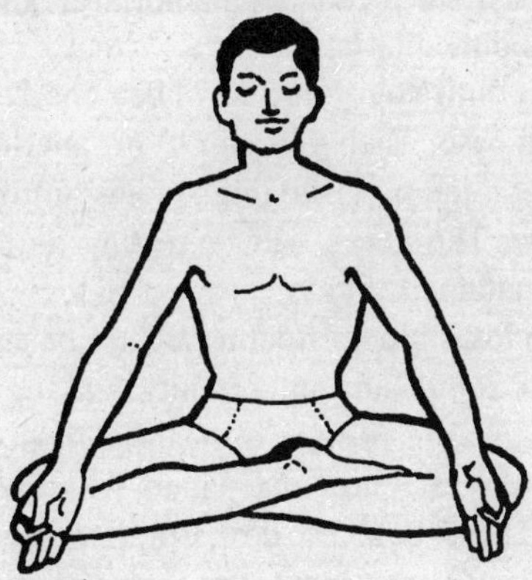

Fig. 24

should be near the abdominal wall. The right foot can be placed below, and the left on top for variation.

The Half-Lotus Posture *(Fig. 25)*
Sit as in the Perfect Posture, but instead of inserting the right foot between the left calf and thigh, bring it higher and place it *on* the left thigh, with the sole turned upward as much as possible. The left foot can be placed on the right thigh if preferred, or for variation.

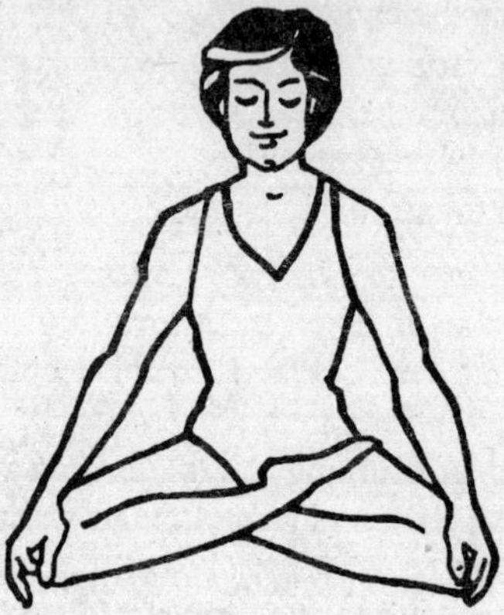

Fig. 25

The Lotus Posture *(Fig. 26)*
Known in Sanskrit as *Padmasana*, this is the seat of the Buddha, and has been used in the East since time immemorial as the ideal posture for sense-withdrawal and meditation.

Do not attempt it until your joints have become flexible enough to do the Half-Lotus with ease. Then you can try to interlock the legs so that each foot is resting on the opposite thigh, soles turning upward as much as your joints allow. The knees will be resting on the floor when true flexibility has been attained.

In the Orient the lotus bloom floating lightly balanced on a still pond is a symbol of peace, composure and serenity, and suggests the inner state of nerves and mind that this posture is meant to induce.

Most adults in the West, particularly men, will find the Lotus difficult to achieve. Some will never be able to do it. But all can learn to sit comfortably and firmly in the Easy Pose, and a good proportion can achieve, with patient practice, the Perfect or Half-Lotus postures.

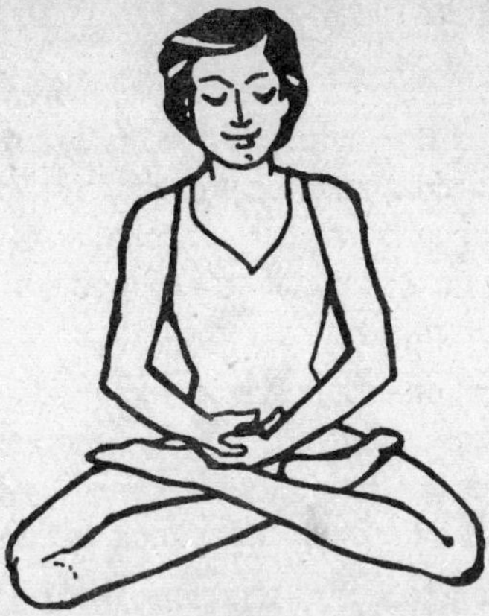

Fig. 26

All cross-legged poses, when thoroughly mastered, give a feeling of balance, calmness and equanimity. Combined with breathing and mental exercises they are of the doorway to the sanctuary of the undivided mind, to the conquest of the ego and environment.

BREATHING AND MENTAL EXERCISES IN SITTING POSES

Sitting in the most advanced cross-legged posture that you can manage, practise one or more of the following exercises.

1. Exhale, turn the consciousness inward, inhale a full yoga breath, hold it for a few seconds while mentally telling the 'inner self' to calm down. Exhale, and repeat six or more times.
2. With the eyes lightly shut, begin taking full yoga breaths; each time you exhale imagine that you are building a cocoon or envelope around your body.

   Feel that this is protecting you from all unwanted outside influences. You are within your cocoon of Peace and Silence. Take from six to twelve breaths in this exercise.

   The psychic envelope you build can become a very real thing with practice – even to the extent of keeping mosquitoes at bay!
3. Find your pulse, or turn the attention inwards and listen to the pulse of your body; breathe to the rhythm of its beat, practising *pranayama* as described in Chapter IV.

PRACTICE FOR THE BUSY STUDENT

You have been practising the limbering-up, breathing and balancing exercises for a few weeks, and are now making a start on the more difficult postures. These will need a good deal of practice, but much of it can be done while you are engaged in other occupations or resting.

1. Instead of sitting on a chair, sit cross-legged on the carpet whenever the opportunity offers.
2. When you must sit on a chair, bring one of your legs up and tuck the foot in with the sole against the thigh – shoe off, of course. After a while change legs. As flexibility increases, try sitting with both feet up, cross-legged, on the chair for as long as you can manage.
3. In bed before going to sleep, bring one foot up with the sole as high as possible against the inside of the opposite thigh. When the ache becomes too much, change legs.
4. As a child you probably succeeded in bringing your big toe to your mouth. Try now to raise it to your forehead before getting into bed. Persist until you succeed.
5. In the quietude of your home, practise all the exercises and postures of this chapter at least three times a week.

As well as advancing you in sense, nerve and mind control, the sitting poses concentrate and balance the currents of the body, bring flexibility to important joints – offsetting the bad effects of advancing years – and prepare you for the higher reaches of yoga.

CHAPTER NINE

Invert Yourself and Stay Young

Man has never ceased in his search for the Fountain of Youth. Just as the old travellers like Columbus hoped to find it beyond the far horizons, and alchemists tried to create the elusive Elixir in their fiery crucibles, so today research scientists throughout the world are seeking it in hundreds of laboratories devoted entirely to this purpose.

From work done already, scientists have decided that the body has no built-in biological 'clock', set by the laws of heredity to stop at a certain time. They have found, for instance, that the life-span of certain animals can be increased enormously through changes in nutrition patterns, the feeding of anti-oxidants and particular hormones – those powerful substances produced by the endocrine glands.

Working on the long-term study of people, they are deciding that many of the ills of later years are only the delayed effects of causes that begin in youth. Young people under thirty feel that they can abuse their bodies with all kinds of excesses and get away with it. But they are sowing the seeds, in metabolic disorders and imbalances, of a painful harvest to be reaped later on. Hardening of the arteries, for instance, was generally considered a disease of old age, but it is now known that hardening changes in the arteries can begin in a person's twenties. Indications are, from the extensive research, that human life expectancy will, before long, be increased from the present three-score-years-and-ten to a healthy one hundred years.

Important ingredients in the Elixir of Youth are certain self-help measures. You must, the scientists say, avoid over-eating, take plenty of physical exercise and fresh air, and always keep mentally active.

Yoga has, of course, been teaching this for several thousand years. The yogis have demonstrated that life can have a much longer spring-time than is generally thought. In fact they say that life's spring, when the sap of vitality runs strongly in the body, should extend to the age of seventy-five. After that come the summer and autumn, so that man should really live to be well over a hundred.

In both East and West are to be found men and women who, by living according to sound yogic principles, attain these long spans of youthful age. Charles Henry Arnold, for example, wrote a little book* *110 Years of Youth Through Yoga* in 1939 when he was 110 years old. He was born, and his birth was officially recorded in the register of the Church of Saint George, Bloomsbury, in London, in 1829. He began learning yoga in India in 1852 from Swami Chakrananda who was at that time 147 years old.

Another man, born three years earlier than Arnold, was the Shiva Puri Baba, a sage and hermit who spent the last years of his life in the mountains of Nepal near the Tibetan border. His life had followed a strange pattern. The first half century was spent in training and meditation in the remote Himalayas. Then, at the age of 50, he set off to travel the world. He took forty years on this venture – much of which was done on foot. He reached England in the 1890s and became an adviser to Queen Victoria, living near her at Frogmore Cottage in Windsor. After her death at the end of the century, he continued his interrupted journey around the world, and returned to India at the outbreak of the world war in 1914. He again went into seclusion in his remote mountain retreat.

There, in the latter years, he received genuine seekers of Truth. A visitor who talked with him in 1961 – author and scientist John Godolphin Bennett – reported that the sage's eyesight and hearing were perfect, his teeth were sound and gleaming white, his movements had the 'vitality and gracefulness of a child' and he radiated peace and wisdom. One of the secrets of long and healthy living was, the Shiva Puri Baba told him, to know your own body and its needs; you must give it just what it requires – no more, no less. You must know, for example, how much to eat, how much to sleep, how much you can use your mind and how hard you can work. This is all good yoga.

Bennett, who saw him not long before he died at the age of 137, said that he 'seemed to know all that was going on all over the world, and clearly understood the problems of modern living'.

Apart from such sages, whose great ages can be verified, and whose virility to the end has been witnessed by many, apart from yoga practitioners of the Western World, who seem physically only half their

* Published by Attilla, London, 1939.

chronological years, there are yogis of the East who are said to have reached fantastic ages. Babu Bisudhanan Dhan, for instance, was believed by his pupils to be nearly 300 years old.

Of course, from the personal point of view, not all would elect to have more years in their lives, but is there anyone who would not vote for more life in his years – particularly those latter years? Westernised yoga does not offer the esoteric teachings that will keep you here on this earth plane for several centuries. What it does offer is a chance to enjoy about one century of healthy years – always, of course, within limits set by a Higher Power.

The whole yoga system works towards this age-delaying effect, and it would be wrong to give the credit to one set of postures. Nevertheless, the inverted positions do play a very important part in rejuvenation – and in a way this is not surprising.

For most of our hours we have our feet to the floor and head towards the ceiling, and all that time the force of gravity is tugging at our tissues, working to pull them downwards to the earth. In the lower part of the body the venous blood must climb back to the heart against the gravitational pull; blood to the upper part must be pumped by the heart against the same constant force.

When we invert ourselves we reverse all this. Gravity pulls the tissues, the vital organs, the blood in the opposite direction. We use the attraction of Mother Earth to right the wrongs she has done us by her constant and powerful urge to draw us into her bosom. We balance the forces, and counteract the effects, of too much drag in one direction.

INVERTED POSTURES

The Rocking Chair

This is a good limbering-up exercise to prepare you for the inverted postures.

You are sitting on a rug or blanket, folded to take your full length. Bring your knees up under your chin and interlock your hands securely around your thighs. Breathing naturally, roll backward, and forward; continue the movement backward and forward on your spine and the muscles of your back, like a rocking chair. As flexibility increases you will find yourself going further back onto your neck, but be careful not to do this too soon, otherwise you might strain a muscle. Be content to increase the arc of your movement slowly. Do six to twelve rolls, or continue until you feel you have had enough.

The Plough *(Halasana) (Fig. 27)*

In your last roll in the Rocking Chair exercise, go over slowly, bringing your feet behind your head, and as near to the floor as you can. Maybe they will touch the floor, maybe not. It does not matter; before long you will be resting your toes on the floor with ease, so don't strain for it; enjoy what you are doing.

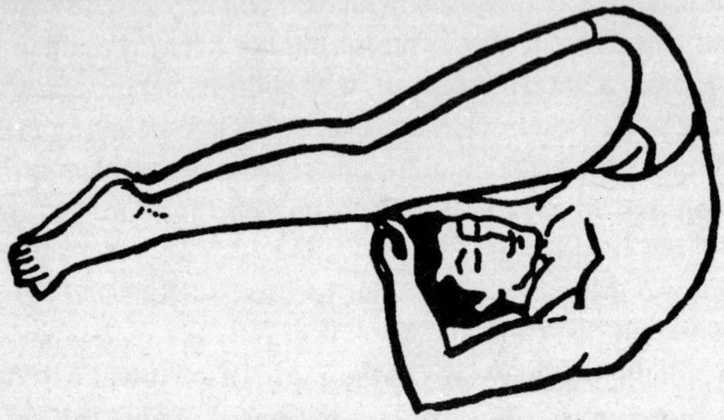

Fig. 27

Place the hands together just above the head, and keep the legs straight. Breathe slowly and concentrate the attention on the upper part of the spine.

At the beginning hold the pose for about ten or fifteen seconds, and then unroll, bringing the feet slowly over and down to the floor. Relax completely.

Variation

Instead of having the hands together just above the head, either stretch the arms above you, resting on the floor, palms up, or stretch them in the opposite direction, palms down.

The Half-Candle *(Fig. 28)*

You will sometimes find this posture under other names, such as the Half-Shoulder Stand and the Reverse Posture.

Execution

Start from the lying position, flat on your back. Swing your legs upward above your head, and support your trunk with the hands at the hips, and elbows on the floor. The trunk is a shallow V-shape, and you are looking straight up at your feet above your face, with some of your weight on your elbows.

Breathe slowly, and as deeply into your abdomen as you can. You will feel some pressure in your face, as extra supplies of blood go into the facial tissues. You can increase the good effects – and offset the discomfort – of this by consciously relaxing the face.

Remain in the pose for about fifteen seconds, or as long as it feels reasonably comfortable. Slowly increase the time until you are holding it with enjoyment for five minutes or more.

Always bring the feet down slowly, and relax after the posture. For full pleasure and benefit, after relaxing the face, consciously relax the whole body in the posture, except, of course, the muscles required to hold you in position.

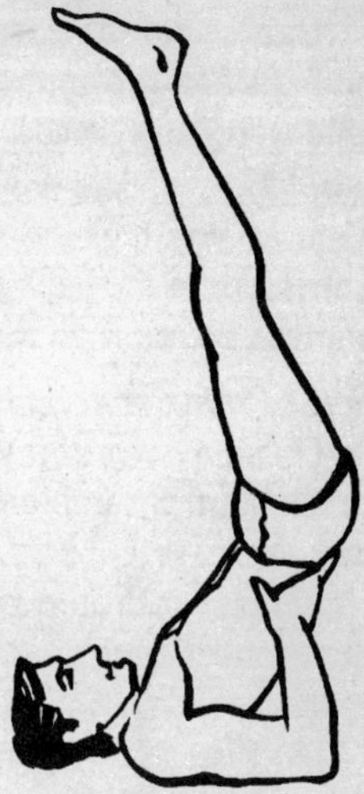

Fig. 28

Comment

If you find it difficult to get into this pose, begin by using a chair or stool to support your body for a few minutes each day. As you get used to the inverted posture, and muscles strengthen, you will be able to do without the support.

The Sanskrit name for the *asana* is *Viparita-Karani* – *Viparita* meaning 'reverse' and *Karani* 'effect'. This implies – by reversing the effects of earth and cosmic forces – the reversal of the wheel of time, and a return to youthful vitality. It is often called the posture of eternal youth.

The Candle (Sanskrit, *Sarvangasana*) *(Fig. 29)*

After you have made some progress with the Half-Candle and Plough, it is time to try this more advanced posture - one of the most important of the yoga *asanas*.

You begin – as for the Half-Candle – from the position on your back, but instead of stopping half-way up, and supporting the body at the hips, you use your hands to help push the trunk higher until it is as vertical as you can get it, without straining.

The ultimate aim is to have your body rising as straight as a candle from the shoulders, with head and neck lying on the floor at right angles to it. The hands support the back as shown in the illustration, but there should be much more weight on the shoulders than on the arms. The straighter your body the easier this is to achieve.

While in the posture, breathe slowly and deeply so that you see your abdomen rise and fall. Relax face and body as in the Half-Candle. Concentrate on the thyroid gland at the base of the throat – where the posture brings pressure – consciously directing cosmic energy to that centre.

Don't hold the pose long at the beginning – perhaps half a minute; but in time you will be able to remain steadily in the posture for minutes enjoying repose and a special pleasure. As soon as you feel the slightest strain, bend the knees, curve the back and slowly return to your starting position on the floor.

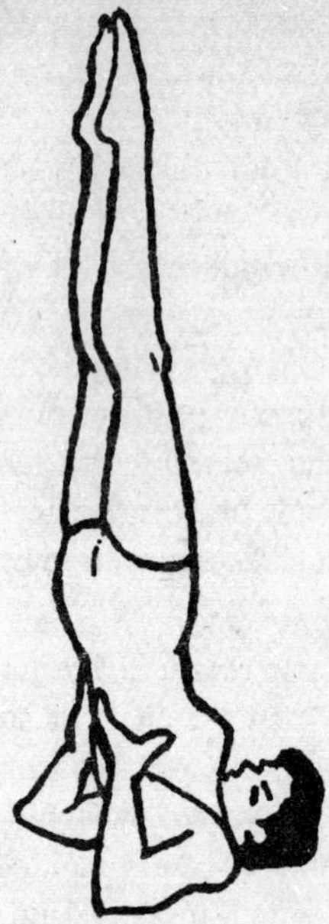

Fig. 29

Some Points on the Posture

(1) Don't worry if you are a very bent candle at the start. Straighten yourself slowly, day by day.

(2) Never drop down like a collapsed pillar at the end. Come down in a controlled, graceful manner.

(3) Instead of returning to the original position from the Candle, you can, as a variation, go over into the Plough, and from there come slowly back to the floor.

(4) Another variation for more advanced students is to take the hands away from supporting the back and raise them vertically above you, parallel with, and in front of the trunk. You are now perfectly balanced on your shoulders and the back of your neck. This pose is called the Balancing Candle.

The Headstand (Sanskrit, *Sirshasana. Sirsh* meaning 'Head')

Being spectacular, this pose has had a great deal of publicity, and is therefore the best-known posture outside yoga circles. Some yoga teachers call it the King of Postures, and all regard it as amongst the most important. But it must be approached with circumspection, and used with moderation.

Phase 1 (Fig. 30 a)

Fold a blanket several times to make a reasonably resilient base. It must still be firm, however, so a pillow, or anything springy like foam rubber, is of no use.

Kneel and join your hands by interlacing the fingers; place the hands and the forearms on the blanket, keeping the elbows not too far apart. Now put the head on the blanket, with its back against the hollow of the locked palms. The head must not, however, be *on* the palms on fingers.

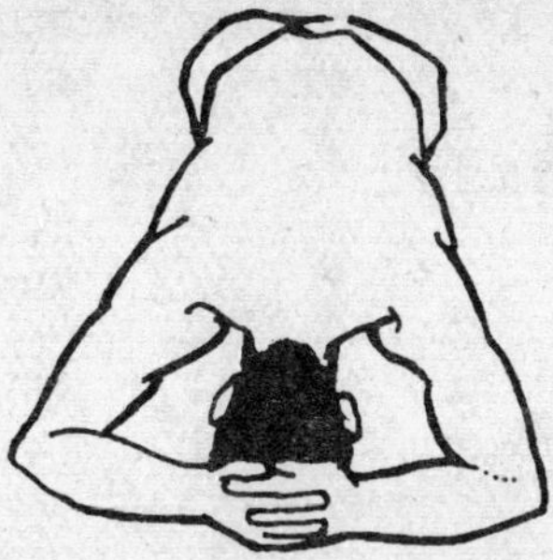

Fig. 30 a

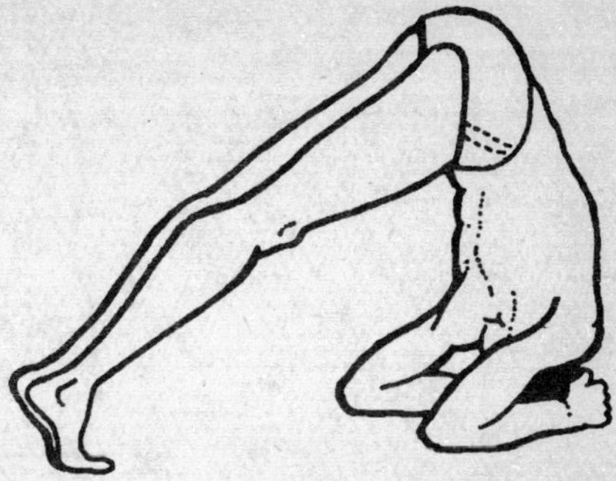

Fig. 30 b

Phase 2 (Fig. 30 b)

Rise up on your toes, and remain a few seconds with weight on head and toes, breathing slowly and deeply. Now the feet must take several steps towards the head.

Phase 3 (Fig. 30 c)

Raise the legs from the floor, bringing the trunk vertical, from head to buttocks; the knees are bent in front of the body. Pause in this pose, breathing evenly and getting a secure balance.

Phase 4 (Fig. 30 d)

Mentally picture yourself upright, with your legs straight above you, and then slowly push the legs up to fit the mental picture. Keep the legs

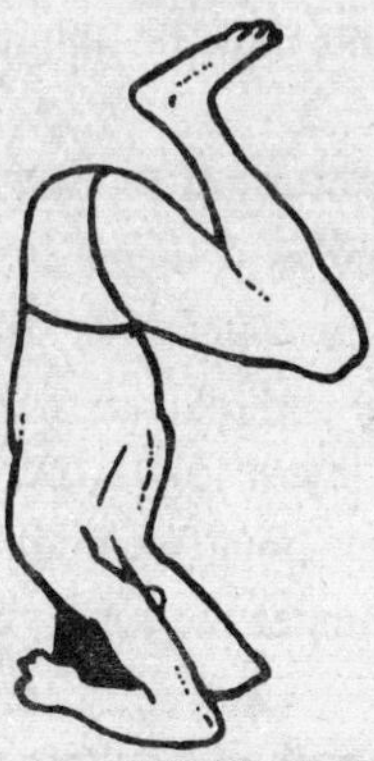

Fig. 30 c

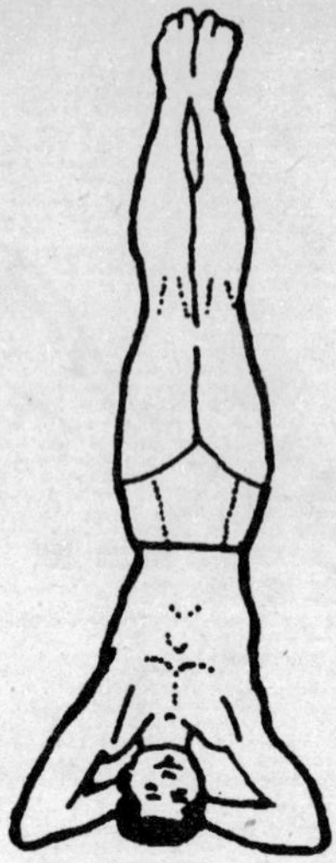

Fig. 30 d

together and point the toes to the ceiling. Breathing is deep and slow; the weight is on the triangle made by your elbows, forearms, hands and head. Any tendency to sway is corrected by muscular pressure at the appropriate points of the triangle.

Conclusion

Bend the knees and bring the feet slowly down to the floor. Rest for a few moments on the knees with the head resting on the hands. Lift your head and sit back on your heels, while you take a few deep breaths and allow the blood circulation to return to normal. Then get slowly to your feet. Remember that all movements must be unhurried and smooth.

Points to Watch

(1) When vertical, be careful not to arch the back as this will cause tension. Relax the body as far as you can. It will assist you in remaining steady if you mentally picture yourself as still as a statue. This will also help to keep the mind steady and relaxed.

(2) At first stay up only a few seconds. Increase the time very gradually to minutes, but set the limit at about five minutes. Long headstands are for advanced yogis or students under the supervision of a *guru.*

For Beginners

Your main initial problems will be weakness in the muscles, and fear of falling over backwards. To overcome the former, practise each phase until you can do it with confidence, before passing on to the next. To eliminate fear of falling, practise in a corner. Place your head on the floor far enough away from the walls so that, when your body goes up, it will rest snugly in the corner.

After a while you can graduate to one wall instead of a corner. Make your headstand about two feet away from it, so that you can use your feet with your knees bent against the wall to prevent yourself from toppling over backwards, if necessary.

When you acquire the confidence to spurn walls, it may still be a good idea to place a cushion behind you to break the impact of a tumble. Actually, even without a cushion, you will not hurt your back if you relax, curve your trunk, and roll with the fall.

Another idea for a beginner is to ask another person to assist. At Phase 2, the assistant lifts a leg to the upright position, and as the other one follows, he steadies both legs and lightly holds them in place.

Variations

The legs can be moved about and held in different positions while you are in the headstand. They can, for instance, be opened sideways, or one put backward and the other forward as if you are walking, or they can be folded into the Lotus Posture – as in *Fig. 30 e*.

Practice Guidance

The inverted postures should not be practised by people with high blood pressure. If there is any serious organic trouble of any kind, a doctor should be asked for advice before they are attempted.

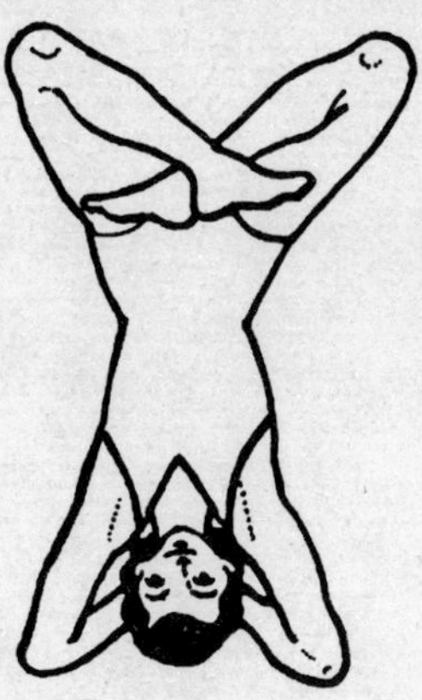

Fig. 30 e

Try to practise these postures every day until you can manage them with comfort and pleasure, after that do them at least three times a week.

Extra Benefits

The health-giving and age-delaying effects of the inverted postures comes not only through using gravity to offset its own damage, but also by reversing the lines of force of earth and cosmic radiations.

All the inverted poses benefit the thyroid gland, and because the endocrine glands are so closely interrelated, all reap rich rewards that are felt throughout the entire system.

The postures keep the spine youthful, nourish the brain, and stimulate the work of vital internal organs. This means in effect that they calm the nerves, drive away any feelings of depression, promote mental energy and work strongly against those bugbears of modern living – constipation and dyspepsia.

When one has advanced some distance on the yoga path, these postures have an additional effect. By bringing extra supplies of blood to the brain, they simulate the dormant psychic centres, and develop powers of extra-sensory perception, such as telepathy and clairvoyance. But these by-products of yoga training come only as the yogi progresses spiritually and can use them wisely.

CHAPTER TEN

Bend Backward for Health

The Cobra Posture *(Fig. 31)*
The Sanskrit name is *Bhujangasana – Bhujanga* meaning 'cobra', the Indian snake that raises the upper part of its body at right angles to the ground, as the yoga student endeavours to do in this highly important *asana.*

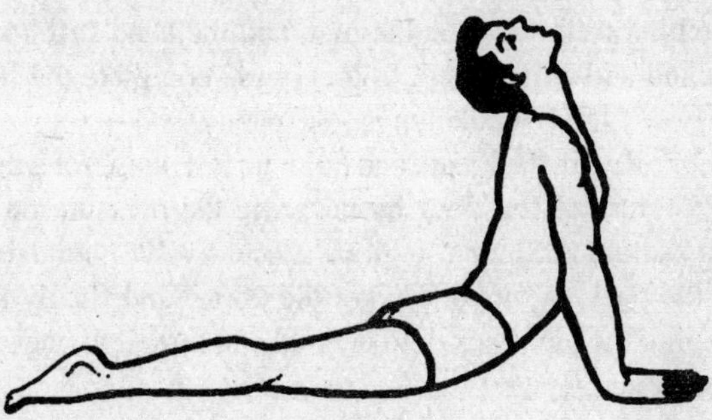

Fig. 31

Execution
Preliminary: Lie face downward on your folded blanket. Place the palms of the hands flat on the blanket under the shoulders, with the tips of the fingers pointing forward. The feet should be together and pointing backward. The face will be turned to one side or the other – cheek on the floor. Relax the whole body with special attention to the feet and legs. Let the breath flow naturally.

The following phases of the posture should flow as one movement.

Cervical Phase: Turn the face forward and slowly raise the chin upward and backward, stretching the throat muscles. Put your consciousness in the upper (cervical) part of the spine. Feel the movement starting in the first vertebra just below the skull and proceeding downward as you bend the head back.

Dorsal Phase: The upward movement continues, raising the chest as far as possible without pressing on the hands. Your attention goes into the dorsal vertebrae, from the region of the neck down towards the waist.

Lumbar Phase: When you have risen as far as possible, using only the back muscles to lift you, exert pressure on the hands to raise the chest still further. At the same time begin to inhale deeply. You will feel the tension moving into the lower back, or region of the lumbar vertebrae. The abdomen should be kept as close to the floor as possible, and the head arched backward as far as it will go. Continue the deep inhalation throughout this and the next phase.

Sacral Phase: Bend the whole spine further back until you feel pressure in its lowest, or the sacral region. Being careful not to strain any muscle, try with gentle pressure to straighten the arms. This will prop your trunk up vertically from the floor.

Keep the hips well down on the mat, and the head still back with the throat stretched and chin raised. In this phase complete the intake of air that should now fill the whole lungs to capacity.

Conclusion: Retain the breath and hold the last phase for a few seconds. Then slowly return to the floor by reducing the pressure on the hands, relaxing the sacral and lumbar regions successively; then using only the muscles of the back as support, lower the dorsal and finally the cervical region, bringing the face back onto the mat and turned to one side. Exhale as you come down.

This completes one cycle of the Cobra. Relax for a while, letting the breath flow naturally, and then repeat the cycle. It can be done three or four times before you move on to another posture.

Variant 1

Instead of pushing the head back, press the chin in to the throat. Otherwise the movements are exactly the same as above.

Variant 2

When you have made progress with the Cobra, try this variant. Carry out the movements in the normal way, but when you have completed the backward bend, bring the head upright on the shoulders, and remain in the pose while you take two or three deep yoga breaths. Make your final exhalation as you return slowly to the floor.

Some Health Benefits

It you keep the consciousness in the back, noting every pressure and enjoying the movement, the Cobra will do wonderful work in keeping the spine supple and straight, and in toning-up the thirty-one pairs of nerves that emanate from the spinal column.

Also it invigorates and strengthens the muscles of the back and abdomen, and has purifying and toning effects on the kidneys, and the adrenal and thyroid glands.

Note: People with hyperfunctioning thyroid glands should not practise this posture.

The Half-Locust Posture *(Fig. 32)*

Sanskrit name: *Ardha Salabhasana.*

Lie flat on the floor on your stomach, hands along the sides, resting easily with the palms up, feet together and toes pointing backwards. The face is turned to one side or the other. Relax completely.

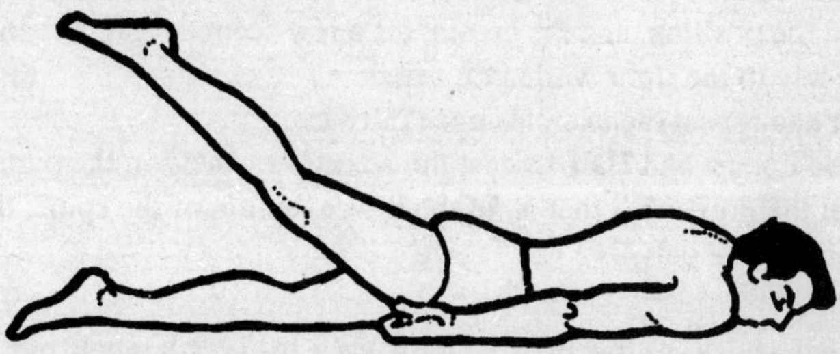

Fig. 32

Take a deep yoga breath, closing the hands lightly, and bringing the face forward with chin on floor. Retain the breath, and raise one of the legs as high as you can, toes pointing backward. Keep the trunk and other leg firmly on the floor. Hold the pose for a few seconds, and then return the leg to the floor while you exhale. Rest and then raise the other leg in the same manner.

Repeat two or three times, and then rest and relax. When you are proficient in the Half-Locust, learn the full Locust.

The Locust *(Fig. 33)*

Sanskrit name: *Salabhasana.*

The starting position is the same as for the Half-Locust.

Close the fists and place them under the hip bones – *on end* so that they give the maximum life to the pelvis.

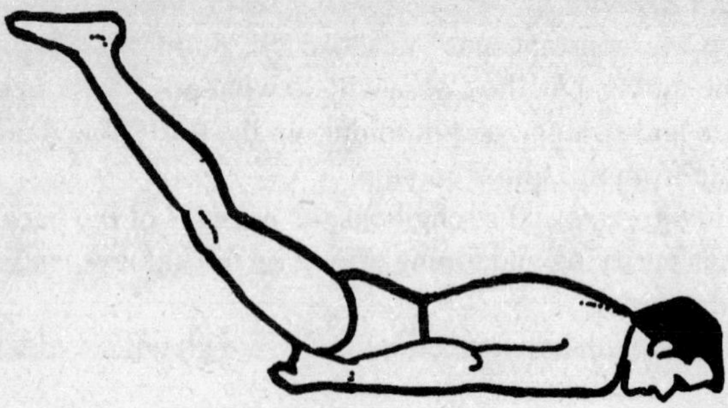

Fig. 33

Take a full yoga breath. Hold it and with face turned forwards raise *both* legs as high as you can manage without straining. Keep them straight and together with the toes pointing backward – just as you would in a good dive into water.

Hold the position, and the breath, for a few seconds and then lower the legs slowly to the floor while you exhale.

Rest and repeat the exercise once or twice.

In the Locust and Half-Locust the attention is held in the parts where you feel the pressure – that is, in the lower section of the spine, the back muscles and the pelvis.

Variation

Perform the posture after an exhalation while the breath is held *out*, instead of in.

Points to Watch

1. Don't strain to achieve a high lift. Most people can raise their feet only a few inches at the beginning. Each time you practise you will go a little higher with enjoyment. Remember it is the effort not the height that brings you the great benefits from this posture.
2. When you have strengthened your back and your mental control sufficiently, you will be able to hold your legs up for a longer period while you take several deep breaths.

Some Benefits

These two *asanas* strengthen the muscles of the back and loins, and help to correct faulty posture. Like the Cobra, they help to cleanse and rejuvenate the kidneys. By acting as a powerful stimulus to the internal organs they are amongst the most effective postures in preventing intestinal trouble and constipation.

The Bow *(Fig. 34)*

Sanskrit name: *Dhanurasana – Dhanur* meaning 'bow'.

Preliminary: Lie on the stomach, relaxed and breathing naturally, hands lying along sides and feet together. Bend the legs, bringing the heels towards the buttocks. Grasp an ankle in each hand.

Phase 1

Take a full breath, and pull on the ankles so that the thighs are lifted off the floor, the chest remaining down against the mat. Hold for a few seconds and let the thighs down as you exhale – but keep hold of the ankles.

Rest for a moment or two, and then after taking another full yoga breath, pull again on the ankles, but this time keep the thighs on the floor, and raise the chest and upper part of the body. Hold for a moment and then bring the chest down, let go the ankles, flatten out on the floor, and relax.

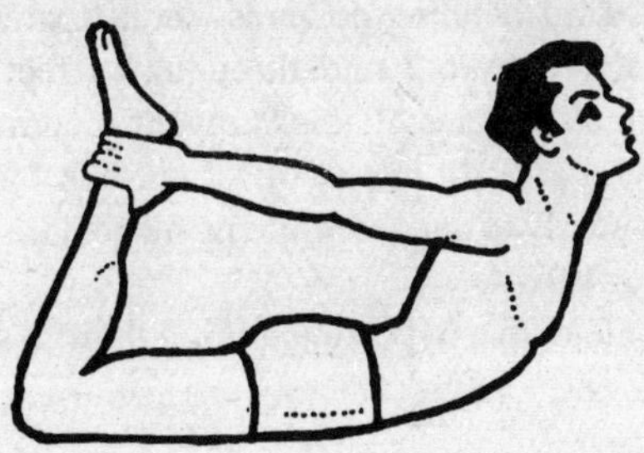

Fig. 34

Repeat, raising the thighs and then the chest several times.

After you have made some progress – perhaps after three or four practice sessions – proceed to:

Phase 2

Take hold of your ankles behind your back as in Phase 1, but now, pulling hard with your arms, raise thighs and chest off the floor *at the same time.* The action is not to pull the legs down towards the back, but to try to straighten the legs against the pull of the arms. The head is held high and the body curves like a bent bow – arms and calves forming the tautened bowstring.

After holding the pose for a few seconds, lower the chest, legs and arms to the floor as you exhale. Rest, breathing deeply and relaxing. Repeat the pose two or three times according to how you feel. Mentally observe all the stretched muscles as you do the exercise.

Variant 1. Reverse the breathing – that is, exhale as you go into the pose and inhale as you come out of it.

Variant 2. Hold the Bow, with the consciousness in the pelvic region, while you take several full yoga breaths; let go and relax on the final exhalation.

Help for Beginners
Owing to stiffness in the back, hips , or knees some beginners find it hard to reach the ankles with the hands. To overcome this handicap they should loop a folded cloth or belt over each foot, holding one in each hand, and pull on those.

Bow Benefits
This posture does wonderful work on the spine, back, abdomen and all organs concerned with these areas. It stimulates the subtle processes in the glands and the invisible functioning of the body's metabolism. Specifically and visibly, it relieves gas, indigestion, sluggishness of liver, and like the other backward-bending postures – constipation. It is very beneficial for an underactive thyroid, and, through its effect on the glands, and also on the abdominal muscles, it helps prevent accumulation of abdominal fat. Anyone who already has a roll of surplus fat on the abdomen, should try rocking gently to and fro while in the posture. This will increase its adipose-reducing effects.

Warning: Anyone with a hyperfunctioning thyroid should not practise this posture.

Practice for odd moments

If you have not done any gymnastics for a long time, your back will probably be as stiff as the trunk of an old tree. You have to get it as supple as a willow branch. We often bend forward in daily activities – to do certain chores, to pick up things – but seldom do we bend backward. Yet the spine and back need such exercise.

Several times a day, whenever you think of it, bend backward, letting your arms go behind you so that your fingers slide down the backs of your thighs. See what point you can reach, and try to improve on it each time until you can touch the backs of your knees, or go even lower.

Another good exercise is to stand with your back to a wall and bend over until you can see the wall. Put your hands against it to help you go further over. When you can kiss the wall you have made excellent progress.

You must use judgement in these exercises and be careful not to strain a muscle. There must be gentle pressure, but no hard forcing.

Will you remember to do these things? If not, it is better to set a certain time for them – say before every meal – during the next few weeks.

When your trunk has become really flexible through these little exercises, you will find the backward-bending postures much easier, much more enjoyable, and much more beneficial.

Remember, don't do the exercises straight after eating anything, and allow three hours after full meals before doing the postures. After you can perform them with ease and comfort, practise these vitally important backward-bending *asanas* at least three times a week.

CHAPTER ELEVEN

Much Can Be Done on Your Knees

The influence of physical posture on man's non-physical aspects – his feelings, attitudes, thoughts – has always been recognised in religious ritual. Kneeling is a posture of prayer in Christianity and also other religions. There is no doubt that it helps to induce feelings of peace and calm, attitudes of humility and submission to a Higher Will.

By lowering our physical stature we can somehow elevate our consciousness, raising it towards the Cosmic Consciousness.

This is the true, the scientific process of prayer – to plug-in, as it were, to that Something which lies above and beyond both mind and body, to submit our faulty lower natures to its benign influence. In this gesture words are not necessary, though they sometimes help to create the right feelings within ourselves. This elevation of our consciousness is the only thing that can really change us.

There is a common saying that human nature cannot be changed. But it *can* be; it is, in fact, continually being changed, and this upward reach of consciousness is the catalyst that brings about the change.

Through it man opens himself to the great Cosmic Influence as a lotus bloom opens itself to the sunshine. While this can be achieved from many postures of the body, there is no doubt that certain traditional postures do help. These are the cross-legged and the kneeling positions.

Both types are valuable and both should be practised, but some people find more immediate effects from the kneeling posture. After a few moments in the pose they find themselves invaded by an atmosphere of peace, calm and upliftment. The effects, as in all yoga *asanas,* are, of course, on man's three aspects – body, mind and soul. The energies in the body are stabilised and balanced, the mind is calmed and the spirit uplifted.

Exercises and *asanas* on the knees play an important part in the yoga alchemy that transmutes the base metal of man's lower nature into the gold of a complete, remade human being.

Kneeling Posture

Sanskrit name: *Vajrasana*

Kneel, keeping your feet together, your soles turned up and toes pointing backwards. Try to sit on your heels. If you find this difficult, rock backwards and forwards from your hips for a time while sitting back as close to your heels as possible. This will help to relax the tensions, and make your knees and ankles more supple.

With practice the pain will go, and you will be able to enjoy sitting back on your heels. Place the hands on the thighs, with the back of the left hand resting in the palm of the right (or rest them on the knees, palms downwards). Close your eyes, or half-close them, and look steadily at an imaginary point a few inches beyond the tip of your nose.

Breathe slowly, deeply, in the yogic manner. With each inhalation feel that you are drawing the cosmic energy, the *prana,* in through your head; feel it passing through your body stabilising and balancing the forces within. As you breathe out, feel that all impurities leave you and go to earth.

Keep the mind calmly and wholly on these feelings of purification and peace. Hold the posture for several minutes, or until the joints tire.

Note: the deep-breathing and *pranayama* exercises given for the cross-legged postures can be done – and *should* sometimes be done – in this kneeling pose.

The Folded Leaf *(Fig. 35)*

The Sanskrit name for this is *Yoga-Mudra, mudra* meaning 'symbol' or 'gesture.'

From the kneeling posture bring the body slowly forward until it is lying on the thighs, with the forehead on the floor. Slide your arms back

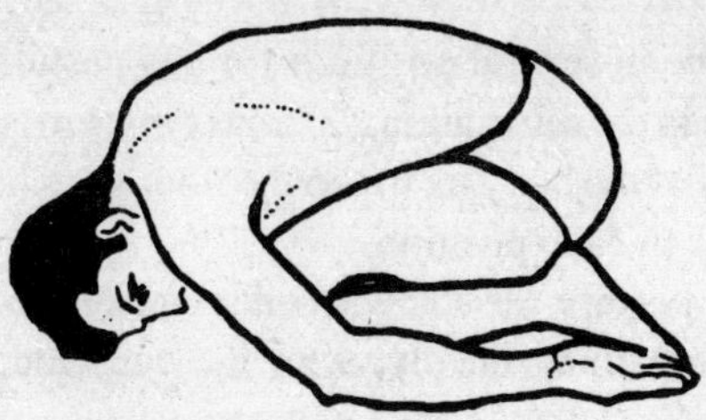

Fig. 35

as you go down, so that they rest on the floor along the sides of the legs, palms facing up.

Your body is now folded in three layers – calves, thighs and chest. At first you will probably feel some pressure in the face. Relax this; relax the whole body; breathe slowly and deeply; remain in the posture until the body and mind feel rested and renewed.

Benefits

You will soon feel the effects of this relaxing posture on the mind and nerves. It is a gesture of obeisance creating an attitude of humility that induces inner calm and refreshment. Physically it tones up the facial tissues.

Full Backward Bend *(Fig. 36 a)*

Sanskrit name: *Supta-vajrasana.*

Kneel, sitting on your heels. Now part the feet and sit between them on the floor, or as near it as you can. Lean gently backward until you touch the floor with one elbow and then the other. (If you find this too difficult you can check your backward movement by holding onto a piece of furniture as you go down.)

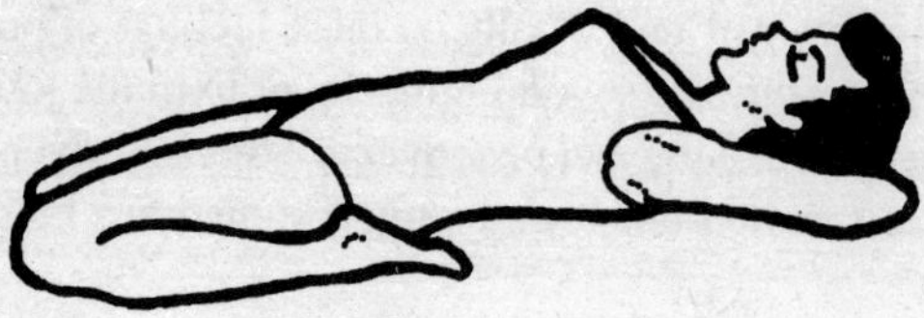

Fig. 36 a

Rest on the two elbows breathing steadily. You may for the first few times be too stiff to go any further back than this, but when you feel able, lower the body onto the floor. This will be easier if you separate the knees a little.

The arms can be in several positions for this posture: (1) hands under the neck as shown in the illustration, (2) arms lying crossed under the back, (3) along the sides of the body, or (4) on the floor stretched above the head. Practise with arms in each position.

Remain in the posture for some seconds (make it some minutes after you are supple) breathing deeply, with the consciousness in the solar plexus.

Return to kneeling posture. Stretch and massage legs.

Variants (Fig. 36 b)
This variation is sometimes called the Thunderbolt Posture. Instead of resting the body flat on the floor, arch the back, shoulders and neck above it, with the crown of the head on the floor and the face looking upside down at the opposite wall. The palms of the hands are placed together in a prayer gesture above the chest – or alternatively the hands hold the calves.

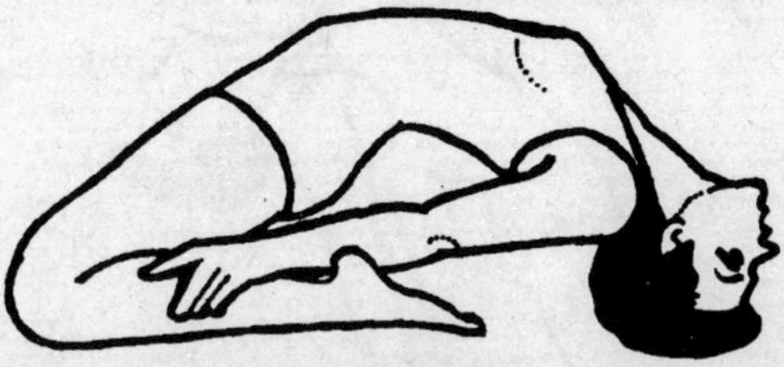

Fig. 36 b

A further variation is to arch the back even more so that the buttocks and thighs are off the floor, and the arch is supported at one end by the head and at the other by the knees and lower legs.

Benefits of the Full Backward Bend
The thighs and abdominal muscles are stretched to the limit, so that these, along with the pelvic organs, spine, and the nerves connected with the sex functions, are strengthened and toned. The posture gives a good neckline, preventing double chins. It also overcomes headaches and the bad effects of too much brain work.

Camel Posture *(Fig. 37 a)*

Sanksrit name: *Ustrasana.*

Phase 1: Assume the kneeling pose, sitting on the heels. Rise off your heels until your body is vertical from the knees up. You are standing on your knees. Place the palms together in front of the body in the gesture of prayer. Close eyes and breathe deeply a few times.

Phase 2: Inhaling deeply, retain the breath and bend over backwards as far as you can. Straighten up to the vertical position\, as you exhale. Do this two or three times.

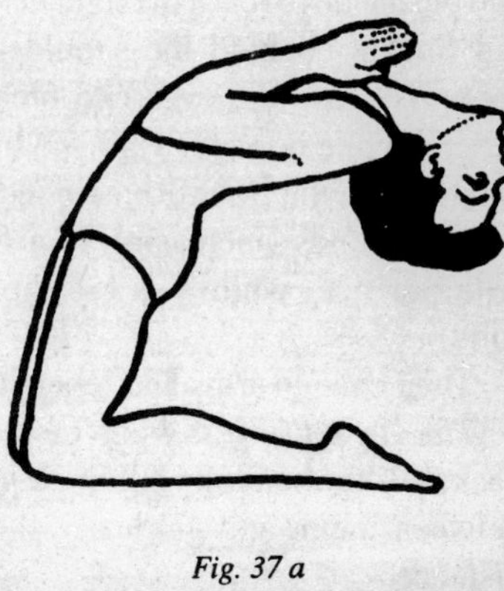

Fig. 37 a

Phase 3 (Fig. 37 b): Inhale and bend right over backwards, placing the hands on the ankles. Remain for a while in this position, body in a graceful curve and head well back. Breathe deeply. Mentally note all the points of tension. Relax the body, except for the muscles necessary to hold the pose.

Finally, straighten up, then sit back on the heels; calm the heart and inner self with rhythmic breathing.

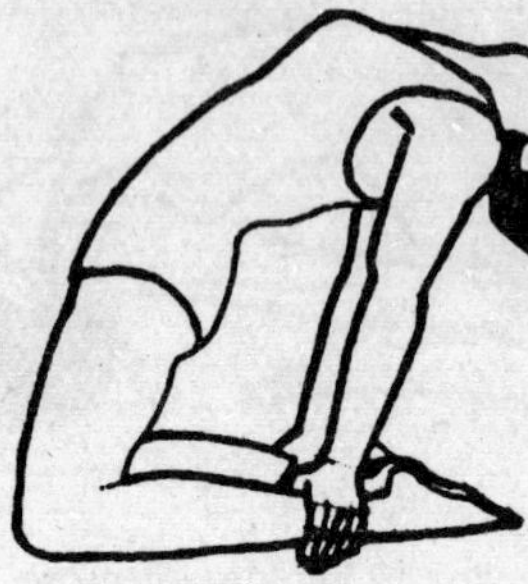

Fig. 37 b

Benefits

The Camel helps to keep the glands functioning properly and beautifies the waistline.

The Grip *(Fig. 38)*

Sanskrit name: *Gomukhasana*

Kneel and sit on the heels. Take the right hand over the head and behind the back as far as it will reach. Put the left hand behind the back and push it up to reach the right hand. Interlock the fingers behind the shoulder blades (as shown). Close the eyes and breathe deeply. After a while bend forward and try to rest the forehead on the floor. Remain in this pose for a few seconds (increasing to a few minutes with practice) while you breathe slowly and fully.

Then change arms and repeat the exercise.

Tip: If your fingers won't meet behind your back, link the hands by holding a handkerchief between them, and gradually shortening the distance.

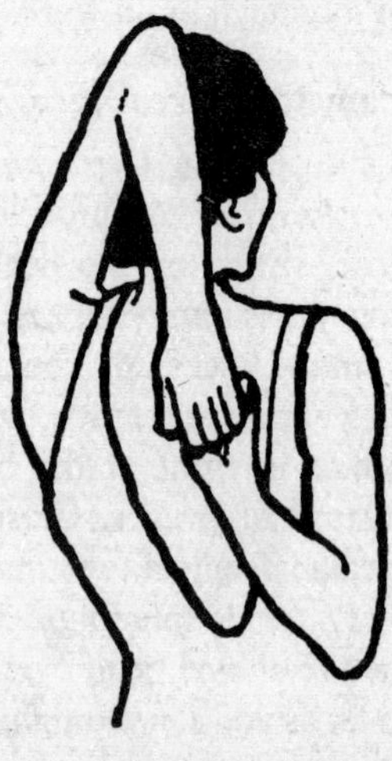

Fig. 38

Benefits
This is one of yoga's 'eternal youth' poses, designed to improve circulation to the facial tissues and prevent wrinkles. It also strengthens the trapezius muscles, keeps the shoulders back and the spine straight.

The Lion Posture *(Fig. 39)*

Sanskrit name: *Simhasana*
Start with the keeling pose, hands on knees, palms downward. Inhale a deep breath; exhale it and at the same time spread out and stiffen the fingers, open the mouth, thrust the tongue out as far as possible and open the eyes wide. The whole body should be tensed and stiff. Hold the pose for several seconds, then relax, and repeat three or four times.

Note: In very bright light keep the eyes closed while in this posture.

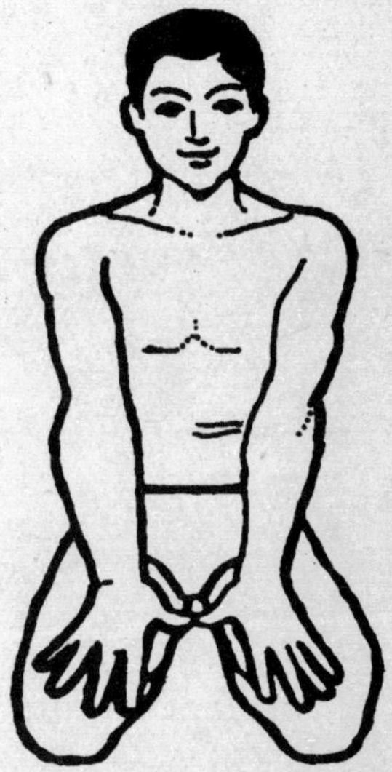

Fig. 39

Benefits
This pose exercises and tones-up, with extra supplies of blood, the muscles of the throat, tongue and neck.

It is more beneficial, yoga adepts believe, if performed in the open, with the mouth turned to the sun, so that the rays enter the throat.

Many yoga students have found that it prevents, relieves, and sometimes quickly cures, a sore throat.

Odd Moment Practice

Do these while watching television or at other odd moments.

(1) Kneel on the floor, sitting on your heels instead of sitting in a chair.

(2) When you are sitting in a chair, rest a leg on the opposite knee, take hold of the foot in one hand and circle it at the ankle. Do about a dozen circles in each direction. Loosen-up both ankles this way.

(3) See how far you can reach each hand up your back between the shoulder blades. Aim to scratch the base of your neck.

(4) Standing on one leg, bend the other and bring the foot up behind you. Take hold of the foot near the toes and try to press it in, flat against the buttocks. This stretches both knee and ankle.

Posture Practice

Practise most of the kneeling postures every day, until you can do them with ease. Then do several of them at least three times a week. You can choose the most convenient time for practice provided it is, as always, three hours after a meal.

CHAPTER TWELVE

Diet—Hygiene—Sleep

Diet

Practical yoga for health and harmony asks that you follow a few simple rules and principles in your eating habits.

The first thing is that you be ruled by true healthy hunger in what you eat and how you eat it, and not by habit, by a false nervous hunger, or by the domination of your palate.

Unfortunately most people are governed to varying degrees by these forces. They are in the habit of eating three meals a day so they must eat them whether they feel truly hungry or not. They have a foolish fear that if a meal is missed they will grow weak or sick. The fact is it's much better to miss a meal if you are feeling heavy in the stomach, 'off colour', or just not hungry. Your stomach will be grateful for the rest. The 'little self' inside you, who likes to follow habits, will feel deprived, of course, but will have to agree that you feel much better for the discipline.

What I have called 'nervous hunger' is closely linked with the fast and furious tempo of modern living. It makes us eat as a kind of escape from pressure, or compensation for overwork and strain on the nerves. It is rather as if that 'small self' in us – like a child – must have its reward for suffering, in sweets and buns.

Nervous hunger not only makes us eat too often, and too much of the wrong things, but it also leads us to eat too fast. How many people fall on their food and devour it like hungry wolves! This way of eating is all right for the wolf; Nature, knowing his needs for speedy, competitive snatching and gobbling in the pack, provided him with a stomach to digest half-masticated food. But man does not have that kind of stomach. He is meant to chew his food slowly, masticate it completely in he mouth, so that it is thoroughly mixed with saliva before it goes down to the stomach.

If he fails in this, he sows the seeds of indigestion, dyspepsia and worse troubles. Observe yourself. Are you a wolf or a human? If you tend towards the wolf as an eater, start the practice of counting your mastications; count forty chews for each mouthful. You will find that the food finally slips down without much need for conscious swallowing, and this is as it should be. Keep up the counting practice until slow eating becomes a habit. The discipline also makes for more silence at meals – another benefit to digestion.

Then, there is the palate. This was meant to be a guide to what is good for us, but under the unnatural conditions of our lives today the palate leads us astray. By nature it likes sweet things, so that it led primitive man to the sweet, good, vitamin-producing fruits. In modern life it takes us to the sugars, the cakes, the chocolates, the sweet desserts. It can't have enough of these; but, of course, the stomach, the blood, and the rest of the system can very soon have too much. As a Dictator of the State of the body, the palate will bring chaos, disease, unrest and eventual ruin.

Moderation is the law here as elsewhere in yoga. You must use judgement, discrimination, will-power. In quantity probably fifty per cent of what you eat is indulgence rather than appetite. On the question of quality, you are most likely eating too many sugary foods, cakes, sweets, fats and starchy foods. These are the weight increasers.

Take more fresh fruit, fruit juices, fresh salads, nuts; learn to like yoghurt and buttermilk, eat more protein food, such as cheese, eggs, vegetables (preferably uncooked or steamed). Unless you want to increase your weight, substitute honey for sugar wherever possible.

Yoga does not ask you to be a vegetarian, but suggests that you decide to eat less meat until you stop eating it altogether. While yoga does not insist that you become a teetotaller, it certainly requires that the drinking of alcohol should be done in moderation.

The finest beverage of all is water – it flushes the kidneys, cleanses the blood, clears the complexion and carries the poisons out of the system. Seventy per cent of your body is water, and losses must be replaced. The yoga student should drink at least two pints of pure water per day and preferably more.

In brief, yoga's advice on the matter of diet is – 'Eat less, eat more slowly, eat more fresh foods and less sugars, starches and fats than is usual in the diet. Instead of white bread eat wholemeal bread which retains more of the grain's valuable minerals and vitamins. Eat for health and it will bring you more joy in the end than if you eat for the sake of indulgence.'

Yoga exercises will develop the discrimination, and the inclination, to help you understand and attain the right balance of foods for your individual needs. They will also help you to realise that for man eating is something more than just an instinctive act. Forms of life – animal or vegetable or both – have been sacrificed in order that you may eat. The sacrifice is not only to serve the needs of your physical vehicle but, through that, your mind and your true spiritual self.

Rituals of the ancient religions implied this inner truth. Life sacrificed was offered as food to the gods, which had an inner as well as an outward meaning. The inner or esoteric meaning was that the fruits of the earth are to serve the Divine Life that lies within the body, as well as beyond it.

Remembering this deep truth, we should eat our food in meditative mood, in humble thanksgiving, and in silence – as far as can be. Certainly, we should never eat in an atmosphere of debate, bickering and emotional upset.

Fasting

The modern yoga student should make some use of this powerful instrument of ancient traditional yoga. Without supervision and expert advice he must not, of course, embark on the long fasts used for the higher yogic purposes.

But he can gain great health benefits, as well as developing his control over the body forces, by practising one-day, two-day, or even three-day fasts. During the fast he should take nothing but water or orange juice (mixed with honey if he feels any weakness).

At first it is wise to choose a time when you have little or nothing to do. Spend a good part of it in bed or lying down and taking life easy. If you have a day of silence at the same time, it will enhance the good effects of the fast.

When you have had some practice in fasting, you could carry out light work, not involving much physical effort, during a one-day fast.

After the fast be careful to start eating with great control as regards both quantity and speed. Break the fast gently with a small meal.

Fasts help to clear the system of toxins and waste products and make you feel really alive. They can be used to cure mild complaints, such as the common cold, indigestion, and other stomach ailments.

Smoking

Just do NOT smoke. If you are already smoking, stop it immediately. No bad harmful habit such as smoking should be stronger than the trained Will of the yoga student.

After you have practised yoga breathing for a time, and begun to visualise and value your lungs, you will not want them blackened, clogged, irritated by smoke and tobacco tars. You will not want your coronary arteries constricted by nicotine. You will not invite cancer of the lungs or throat!

Sense-control will strengthen you to rise above the power of habit and desire. More specifically, if you wish, you can use deep yoga relaxation, like self-hypnosis, to train your subconscious through suggestion. When profoundly relaxed, speak to it in a positive way. You may say, for instance, several times – 'There will be no more desire to smoke,' and then, 'When I think of reaching for a cigarette I will shake both hands loosely instead.' Then, during the day, make this relaxing gesture whenever your hands creep towards your pocket for the cigarette packet. Do the auto-suggestion in deep relaxation every day – *twice* a day if necessary. It is the direct road to breaking this and any other foolish or harmful habit.

I know from my own experience, and from that of other yogis and yoginis, that by these methods the controls can be wheedled from the grip of Pilot Nicotine – without undue shock to the psychophysical mechanisms.

Personal Hygiene

Some social historians give Beau Brummell the credit for starting the fashion of the daily bath. In any case it is a fairly recent custom of the West that is still far from being universal. Regular teeth cleaning, encouraged by toothpaste advertising, is general nowadays, though not *thorough*, judging by the thriving dental profession.

And that, with the occasional hair wash, is about as far as we moderns go in the matter of cleansing the body. Thousands of years ago the yogis were teaching their pupils these and several further practices in personal hygiene and purification. Their practices or *kriyas,* as they called them, included the cleaning of the skin, hair, eyes, tongue, teeth, nasal passages, stomach and bowels.

Following the ancient teachings as far as practicable, modern yoga advises the daily bath, or preferably shower. It should not be too hot and, if taken in the morning or during the day, it should be followed by a cold shower. This is, of course, not easy until you are used to it; so educate yourself through stages of tepid showers and cool showers. Learn to consciously relax during the cold shower, and you will learn to enjoy it.

An alternative invigorating morning practice is the cold friction bath. For this you take a rough face-cloth or small coarse towel, dip it in cold water (tepid water until you toughen-up), wring it out as far as need be, and rub your body vigorously. After plenty of hard rubbing, dry off with a soft towel. This should be carried out in a warm place, and if you have any feeling of chilliness, treat only part of your body to the friction bath. Then gradually include more of it until you are able to do the whole physique, back as well, before drying yourself.

If you prefer a cold shower to a cold friction bath, provide the highly-beneficial friction by drying and rubbing yourself down thoroughly with a rough towel. Of course, you must adjust the friction to the quality of your skin; some skins can take plenty of rubbing – others soon become sore.

The cold and the friction together tone-up the circulation in the skin, driving the blood from the vessels and bringing it back again vigorously, so that you feel a warm pleasant glow. In this way the heart is assisted in its work, circulation is improved, the skin is kept healthy and radiant, and you are much less likely to catch the common cold.

Occasional baths to be enjoyed are the oil bath, and the air bath. The oil bath is used whenever the skin appears to be too dry, and also at changes of the seasons – at the end of winter and the end of summer. Following a warm-water bath, rub your body all over with warm oil. Rub the oil well into the skin and wipe off any surplus oil before dressing.

Air baths are always good when the temperature is suitable. Try to take them in the nude; and although indoors with open windows is good, outdoors is even better. Take an air bath whenever practicable, even if it is only for a few minutes. Relax when taking them and feel your skin absorbing the refreshing life-giving properties of the air and *prana.*

Tongue: An old tooth-brush, not too hard, is good for this. Gently rub the tongue clean with it – using plenty of rinsing water – every day.

Nasal passages: The nostrils filter dirt particles from the air every time you breathe. Help their good work by cleaning them out once a week. The easiest way is to breathe warm saline from a bowl through the nostrils and bring it out of the mouth. Make sure that both nostrils are cleansed. Some people prefer to use an eye-bath instead of a bowl in order to cleanse one nostril at a time.

The yogis also use the opposite action. That is, they take water through the mouth and eject it through the nostrils. This is a good purifying practice if you can learn to do it.

Throat: Follow the nostril cleansing by gargling the throat with warm saline – water containing half to a level teaspoon of common salt dissolved in each pint.

Eyes: With slightly warm mild saline wash the eyes several times a week. Use an eyebath, tip the head well back, open the eye and blink several times, so that the saline cleanses the eyeball thoroughly. Cold, instead of tepid, saline may be used if preferred.

This washes away the dangerous dust particles that harbour germs, at the same time refreshing and brightening tired eyes.

Stomach and bowel cleansing: Disciples in yoga *ashrams* of the East learn several traditional techniques for cleansing the stomach and bowels, such as drawing water into the bowels through the anus. These practices involve well-developed conscious control of certain involuntary muscles. Instead the Western student can substitute the occasional – but not too frequent – use of saline enemas and colonic irrigations for cleansing the bowels.

Sleep and Insomnia

There are many degrees of sleep from the shallow to the very deep. Scientific instruments show that during most of it our brains and nerves are not completely in a state of rest. Brain action takes the form of dreams, some of which we remember, but there are undoubtedly many others that we never recall. Most dreams are worrying, frightening or strongly charged with emotion in some way. They set up stresses in the nerves and muscles, and can cause a great expenditure of energy, so that we wake up in the morning feeling worn out instead of rested.

One of the main purposes of sleep is to recharge the body and mind with energy. If our sleep is filled with strain and tensions we defeat this purpose – we expend most, if not all, the energy that comes to us from the great cosmic batteries. How can we correct this?

The answer is to go to sleep as relaxed in body and mind as possible. This can be achieved by pushing your pillow out of the way, lying on your back, and doing the Relaxation Pose (Chapter II), Do it until you are utterly relaxed and light. Then reclaim your pillow, turn on your side, and open yourself to the cosmic energy, the *prana.* Picture this flowing into your body as you glide off to sleep.

This exercise, as well as giving you a truly refreshing sleep, should overcome any tendency to insomnia. However, you may find at any time that you do not slip off quickly while in the relaxed state, but start once more to think about your problems. The psychologist's trick of watching the figures that come behind the closed eyelids, works for some people but not for others. If it does not work for you, you could try *namasmarana*. This means, the repetition of a holy name, preferably one of God's many names. It could be one of the following: Jesus, Rama, God, Krishna, Allah, Sai Baba or a name preferred by the student. It should be short, preferably not more than two or three words such as 'Lord Jesus Christ' or 'Om Sai Ram' or 'Allah Akbar'. It is very important that you choose a name which brings you an inward feeling of elevation. Continue repeating the name silently and if possible picturing at the same time the figure associated with the name. If there is no figure associated with the name in your mind, you could picture something simple such as a light or an object that is pleasing to the mind. If the picture fades, as in time it will, simply go on repeating the name. This practice will empty the mind of thought as you attempt to do in meditation and will at the same time bring an uplift of your spirit. If the repetition of the name does not help you overcome insomnia, try the practice of the English yogi who lived to be one hundred and ten or more, that is, after relaxing completely, be in the most comfortable position and say to yourself 'I am sleepy, very sleepy. I cannot stay awake.'

Appendix

Methods of Application

Perhaps you have read this book through from chapter to chapter as you normally read a book, saying to yourself, 'Yes, the instructions seem easy to follow. I will try them later on.' And now you may be thinking, "Well, there seems an awful lot. I'm so busy, I really doubt if I'll have time for it after all."

But don't be defeated by this negative attitude! Increasing numbers of very busy people – writers, artists, business executives, secretaries, factory workers, housewives – are finding time to do yoga regularly. They discover that it is not an expenditure, but an investment of Time. It does not prevent them doing other things, but enables them to do more through the gifts of greater relaxation, higher levels of vitality, keener concentration, and a more balanced outlook on life.

The way to make the most of the book is this: after reading it through once, go back and practise the exercises chapter by chapter, until you can carry them out without any reference to the text. Get to know all the points about them before you move on to the next set.

Then, after you are familiar with the exercises, begin to plan combinations of them for a full yoga session of anything from half-an-hour to an hour in duration. This is the part that students often find difficult at the beginning.

Here are a few points to help you: Do some deep breathing, some limbering-up and relaxing exercises before starting on the postures. Try to include one or more postures from each of the main groups – kneeling, sitting cross-legged, inverted, bending backward. Always include the Relaxation Pose. At or near the end do some more relaxing, loosening-up, muscle-shaking exercises. Don't be rigid about your programme; if an inner sense tells you that your body needs a certain posture or movement during the session, go into it. This is the kind of inward guidance that you want to develop, and will develop with time and practice. When that time comes, you will not need to plan ahead. You will feel, as you proceed, just what the body should do next, and the session will flow smoothly, pleasantly from beginning to end.

To start you off, here are two suggested programmes.

Programme One

(1) Bending forward – relaxing (Chapter 2, Ex. 2, Fig. 1).
(2) Yoga breathing routine (1) (Chapter 4).
(3) Neck routine (Chapter 5).
(4) Routine for spine (a) (Chapter 5, Fig. 8).
(5) Leg work (1) (Chapter 6, fig. 12).
(6) Abdominal exercise (1) (Chapter 6, Fig. 16).
(7) The 'Ha' Breath (Chapter 4).
(8) The Tree Posture (Chapter 7, Figs. 17 and 18).
(9) Uddiyana (abdominal contractions) (Chapter 7).
(10) Head-to-knee stretching exercise (Chapter 8, Figs. 21) and (22).
(11) Exercises in the Easy Pose, with Posture of Reintegration (Chapter 8, Fig. 23).
(12) The Rocking Chair exercise (Chapter 9).
(13) The Plough (Chapter 9, Fig. 27).
(14) The Candle (Chapter 9, Fig. 29).
(15) The Cobra (Chapter 10, Fig. 31).
(16) The Relaxation Posture (Chapter 2, Fig. 2). (Followed by concentration and meditation in the pose).
(17) Exercises for loosening arms and legs (Chapter 5).
(18) The Headstand (Chapter 9, 30a, b, c & d).

Programme Two

(1) Dropping arms and head – relaxing (Chapter 2, Ex. 1).
(2) Yoga breathing routine (2) (Chapter 4).
(3) Routine for spine (b and c) (Chapter 5).
(4) Leg work – 2 (a and b) (Chapter 6, Fig. 13).
(5) Arm, back, and chest work (Chapter 6, Figs. 14 and 15).
(6) The Whistle Breath (Chapter 4).
(7) The Corkscrew (Chapter 7, Fig. 19).
(8) Spine stretching exercise (Chapter 7).
(9) The Deep Obeisance (Chapter 5, Fig. 11).

(10) The Kneeling Posture (Chapter 11).
(11) The Folded Leaf (Chapter 11, Fig. 35).
(12) The Full Backward Bend (Chapter 11, Fig. 36a).
(13) The Perfect Posture (Chapter 8, fig. 24).
(14) While in the Perfect Pose do *pranayama* exercises (Chapter 4),
(15) Abdominal exercise (2) (Chapter 6).
(16) The Half-Candle (Chapter 9, Fig. 28).
(17) The Bow (Chapter 10, Fig. 34).
(18) The Headstand (Chapter 9, 30a, b, c & d).
(19) The Relaxation Posture (Chapter 2).
(20) Meditation exercise in a cross-legged pose (Appendix).
(21) Exercises for loosening-up arms and legs (Chapter 5).

Exercises for Odd Moments

After you have practised, and know well, the odd-moments exercises given in the various chapters, select several at the beginning of each day for your daily practice. Do them for a few seconds whenever you remember or opportunity offers – when, for example, walking, watching TV, pausing at your desk for a break in your work, after you have finished a chore in the house or workshop.

Here are some eye exercises that should be done at least once a day. They can be performed sitting in the bus or train, at your desk just before you start work, or at any other time that you find suitable.

Eye Exercises

(1) Look straight ahead, then turn the eyes as far as you can to the right, and to the left. Don't move them too quickly; look definitely at a point on the far right and the far left. Make three or four movements in each direction. Close the eyes and rest them.
(2) Do the same, looking up and down instead of left and right. Close and rest the eyes.
(3) Circle the eyes slowly – three or four times in each direction. Then close and rest.
(4) Hold a finger about a foot in front of your eyes. Look at the finger and then at a distant point, and then at your finger again. Do this movement from six to twelve times. Then close the eyes and rest them. This exercise should also be done with the finger held closer to the tip of the nose.
(5) Do Exercise 4 with one eye at a time, holding the palm of the hand loosely over the other eye to block its vision. Close and rest the eyes.

(6) Select a small, very simple thing, such as a knob or a dot on the wall, some distance away. Your eyes should be able to see the whole of the object without moving. Hold the gaze steadily, without staring hard, on the object. Do not blink, and try not to focus too strongly; the eyes should be relaxed as much as possible. When they grow tired or begin to water, finish the exercise by blinking strongly and vigorously several times.

Finally close the eyes and stroke the eye-lids gently with your finger-tips, feeling that you are wiping away all tension and all impurities. Make a cup of the palms, learn forward and put the cup over the eyes so that no light comes in. Do not press the hands against the eyeballs. Relax the eyes completely in this way for several minutes.

Exercising the Mind

The last eye exercise of the list helps to make the mind steady. Hatha yoga works, as we said earlier, on the body, and also on the mind *through* the body. But as taught today, it usually includes as well some exercises that work directly on the mind – some elementary Rajah yoga.

These exercises aim at developing concentration, and higher levels of consciousness through meditation and contemplation.

A large part of our school education is aimed at teaching us to concentrate on certain subjects. But yoga aims at a more pin-pointed concentration than this. The mind, which is normally scattered, to an extent, throughout the senses, must be gathered together at a single point and held there. To assist this, an object may be chosen. At the beginning it should be a simple one – perhaps a flower, a sea-shell, a pearl, a candle flame, a piece of fruit or a cross. The actual object may sometimes be used and observed but the general practice is to hold a mental image of it, with the eyes closed. All other images or thoughts must be excluded.

The mind will itself begin to meditate on the object, thinking about its various qualities, its colour, shape, smell, and so on. But soon – following the Law of Association – the mind will want to wander off onto related objects until, having started with a rose, you will perhaps, for example, find yourself thinking about someone you met on your last holiday.

This is just reverie, and no use to your purpose. so you must keep close watch, and bring the mind back as soon as it begins to move off along that chain of associated ideas. Keep it concentrated on the qualities of the rose. Then go a step further in your meditation. Go to the middle of the rose;

try to understand the *roseness* – the essential something that makes it a rose and nothing else. Try to feel this *roseness...* to become one with the rose.

When you have achieved this, you have moved from meditation to contemplation where there is no longer the seer and the seen, as two separate entities. You have lost for a moment the sense of 'I', and become merged with the object. This state brings a wonderful repose to the ego, to the everyday self. You are getting closer to the realisation of the True Self.

Some Specific Meditation Exercises

(1) Practise this, and the next exercise, in your favourite cross-legged or kneeling posture, or in the Relaxation Pose, after the feeling of weightlessness has been reached. You may also practice this, sitting straight-backed on a chair.

Close the eyes and meditate on a simple object of your choice, as described above. Finally imagine that you are not *you*, but the object on which you have been meditating. See the world from its centre as if you are it.

(2) Close the eyes and imagine a rose in a simple vase standing on a table covered with a cloth – all against a plain pale blue background. Picture the shape and colour of these objects clearly, then remove them one by one – first the table, then the cloth, then the vase so that only the rose remains against the background. Finally remove the rose so that now there is nothing but the plain pale blue background. Hold the mind empty of all but this for a few seconds.

(3) Sitting in a cross-legged pose, let your gaze be neutral – you are looking at *nothing* a few feet in front of your face. Now gather the light that is scattered within you and bring it to a point. Project it in front of you so that you see it as a steady point. Project it in front of you so that you see it as a steady flame. Hold your mind itself as still as a flame in a windless place, quite unruffled by thought, for as long as possible.

(4) In bed at night before sleeping, push the pillow aside, lie flat on your back, relax completely, and meditate on the events of the day. Begin with the last event and go back through them one by one to the day's beginning. Picture yourself doing each thing, and understand what you did and why you did it.

You will probably be fast asleep before you get back to lunch-time. But you will have brought many sensations, impressions, emotions into conscious memory and rationalised them. They will not now come back to disturb your dreams, nor will they create unconscious, irrational urges, fears and worries. You have brought them up and mentally digested them – as a cow chews its cud to get the real good from the food it has swallowed.

In this exercise you are also improving your memory, your power of recall from the preconscious mind. Through its practice you can eventually go back to the very beginnings of life, and – some say – even across the threshold into former existence. It is through remembering past actions – and truly comprehending their import – that we begin to know who and what we really are.

Looking back now over the ground we have covered, we see that the theme, the principle underlying all Hatha yoga practice is that these ancient exercises are physical-cum-mental, and that both the mind and the body are themselves only instruments of a Higher Self.

Keep in mind always that the aim of yoga is to make them perfect instruments – worthy, ever-obedient servants. But for this they must be respected and valued. As a modern professor of physical education, and doctor of philosophy, points out, the Higher. Self – or Spirit – does not reach its mastery through abusing or neglecting the body and mind, through violating the laws of healthy living (which is the erroneous view of some ascetics). He says, 'Only a lofty bodily ideal is able, by its beauty and greatness, to cause the necessary enthusiasm to spring from the depths of the soul for the body to find health, strength, beauty, delight in living, spiritualisation, and ascent towards God.' [1]

Yoga is for the Christian West as well as for the East. You do not need a knowledge of Hindu philosophy or religion in order to practise it, for – as a Christian yogi monk writes – Men in all places are men, and to reach a higher aim, to live according to the spirit – in whatever sense this may be understood – they have to get over the same obstacles, face the same difficulties, and avoid the same snares...

'Help yourself and heaven will help you. Nothing could be simpler, nothing could be wiser.'[2]

---

1 Max Marin, *l'Athlete chretien, Comment le former* (Presses de Belgique, Brussels).

2 J.M. Dechanet, O.S.B., *Christian Yoga* (Burns and Oates, London).

Postscript

There is no doubt whatsoever that if you do the exercises in this book regularly and faithfully you will gain great benefits in health, vitality and well-being. You will also, commensurate with the Higher will, enjoy a longer life. This is not the aim of yoga, in spite of this worthwhile achievement, as there is a higher goal to be reached. And that is the union of your everyday self or ego with a higher Self. This Self with which we can find ultimate union goes under many names such as the divine spark, the God within, man's true identity and so on. It is, in fact, the Reality which all human beings are seeking. This is the goal and purpose of human life. We may or we may not be consciously aware of it. There are some *Hatha Yoga* gurus who claim that this ultimate aim can be achieved through the practice of *Hatha Yoga* itself. Others state that the purpose of *Hatha Yoga* is to bring the body and mind of the individual to a state of purity and strength that will act as a firm foundation. This in turn will act as a kind of landing pad for the great Enlightenment or Self-realisation when it finally comes. Otherwise, the gurus maintain, the individual may be overcome and completely undone by the great experience.

After reaching a certain stage in *Hatha Yoga* practice, you may, like many others I have known, want to know something about the pathways of the so-called higher yogas. Therefore I give a brief introduction to them here. While there are many winding tracks leading up the mountainside of spiritual endeavour, there are four main pathways that will take the seeker of Truth right up to the summit of the mountain, right to the glorious achievement of life's endeavours. You may yourself feel inclined towards one of these paths due to your tastes and temperament. Yet ultimately it will be your *karmic* needs that will decide the best path for you.

One of the four pathways is the *Rajah Yoga*, which has been mentioned earlier in this book. This yoga of the mind and its complete control seems to grow naturally out of the yoga of the body and mind that we call *Hatha Yoga*. Many *Hatha Yogis* at first feel inclined towards this particular higher yoga. But with its stern disciplines for the thinking mind, the emotional mind and the lower propensities, as well as its strict lifestyle, it becomes a highly disciplined way of life. Therefore, *Rajah Yoga* can be likened to a steep, stiff climb up the mountainside. It can be said to be the path for the few rather than for the many. Yet, at their less rigorous levels, the disciplines of *Rajah Yoga* can be a help on the other pathways.

The second of the main four pathways is the yoga of knowledge – also known as the *Jnana Yoga*. This is for the deep and serious student; one whose mind and heart find joy and satisfaction in the continual search for Truth at all levels. The danger on this pathway is that it may lead to a dead-end. The student, thinking that he can reach his goal through his mind and intellect, develops too much mental pride and too much individual ego and becomes lost in the pleasant scenery of the mountainside. His great error is in thinking that mental study and the intellect can take him to ultimate enlightenment. His learning must bring him the wisdom to realise that he must break through his mental bonds and reach a level beyond his mind in order to find that higher union that he seeks. Like *Rajah Yoga* this is the pathway for only a few individuals. Yet, with the understanding that it brings, it is a necessary aid to the climbers on the other yoga pathways.

A suitable yogic pathway for many people living in the world today is the pathway known as *Karma Yoga*, or the way of work. It is natural for the human being to engage in action – mental and physical. The motive for his action is the vital consideration on this pathway. In childhood his only motive is pleasure and we call this action play. As he reaches adulthood his actions become more organised and directed and we call it work. Now his necessary motivation is to earn a living for himself and for his family. Many will want to do more than just earn enough money for making a living. They will aim at making a great deal of wealth, thinking that this will bring them the satisfaction and happiness that they seek. But the truth is that neither wealth nor the power that wealth often brings will bring happiness and satisfaction to the human being. On the contrary, it will bind the individual more strongly and securely to the world of desire where pain and sorrow outweigh fleeting pleasures. What, then, is the true yoga of work? What is the secret in action that leads not into the impenetrable forest of desires and attachment, but steadily up a clear pathway to the top? Put quite simply it is work done, or action taken, with no thought for the fruits of that action or that work. In Sanskrit this is called *nishkamakarma* or desireless action. If the yogi still has to earn a living, as most do, he will not regard his work for this as the main work of his life. What, then, are the motives for his main actions or work? Perhaps the motive will be duty. Better still if it is duty with the higher love. As he progresses, the thought of duty will lessen and disappear while selfless love becomes his main and only motive. Love of what, you ask? Certainly not of wealth or power or glory of any kind. It will probably be love of humanity and for this great love of his fellow men he must see God in all beings. With this motivation of goodwill towards all men and deep love for all life, he is on this third, but by no means least of the great pathways up the mountain.

The fourth pathway is called *Bhakti Yoga* or the yoga of love and devotion. Spurn it not, for the ancient sages say that it is the easiest pathway and the one most likely to succeed in the present age. It seems that in this dark, materialistic age, those who would seek to explore the deeper dimensions need a Divine form to worship. It is better if the Divine form is living today; yet he may have lived in the past and still be worshipped today. One such divine person is Jesus Christ who still inspires love in the human heart and Christianity at its purest belongs to the Bhakti pathway. Other God–men who have awakened love in the hearts of men and still do so, though their forms have long vanished from the earth, are notably Lord Krishna, Chaitanya and many more who are not so well-known. Today, there lives on earth a God-man who through the great outpouring of Divine love opens the hearts of millions throughout the world and raises them on the swelling tide of love towards the human goal. He is Satya Sai Baba. But while he teaches that love is the main pathway of yoga, he also braces it with the wisdom and discipline of other pathways. Studies of scriptures, selfless work in serving humanity, concentration, meditation and contemplation are some of these.

All the great spiritual teachers interlace the various pathways, while Bhakti remains dominant, into a kind of integral yoga. The truth is that no great yoga pathway is, or should be, exclusive in itself. All are in some degree interdependent, and near the top of the mountain all differences are dissolved and all pathways become one.

The earnest yoga student will find good textbooks to help him on whatever yoga pathway he finds his feet on. Where the emphasis is on

Rajah Yoga, for example, there is the ancient textbook called *Patanjali's Yoga Sutras.* For the yoga of devotion, I can recommend another ancient book called Narada's *Bhakti Sutras,* Narada was a great sage of India's distant past who recommended the *Bhakti Marga* (pathway), or the Yoga of Divine love to all, including his brother, Sage Vyasa, who despite the fact that he had produced books of great spiritual wisdom, still found his life empty. It could only be filled, Narada told him, by Divine Love and so Vyasa wrote a great work of devotion to god known as the *Srimad Bhagavatha.* This has been translated into English and should be read by all aspirants of the higher yogas, as should indeed that great scripture of India that deals with all the yogas. This is the *Bhagavad Gita* or the 'Song of God'.

Index

Some Previous Books by the Author

1. *Yoga For Busy People.* Oldbourne Press, London, 1964. Orient Longman, India, 1971.

2. *Hammer on the Mountain* (Biography of Colonel Henry Steel Olcott, co-founder of the Theosophical Society). Quest Books, Wheaton, U.S.A., 1972.
   Yankee Beacon of Buddhist Light (new edition of the above, renamed). Quest Books, Wheaton, U.S.A., 1988.

3. *When Daylight Comes* (Biography of Madame H.P. Blavatsky, co-founder of the Theosophical Society). Quest Books, Wheaton, U.S.A., 1975.

4. *Sai Baba, Man of Miracles.* Frederick Muller, London, 1970. Macmillan India Ltd., India, 1972. Samuel Weiser Inc., U.S.A., 1973. Vrindavanam Books, London, 1984.
   Also translated into and published in 25 foreign languages.

5. *Sai Baba, Avatar.* Birthday Publishing Co., U.S.A., 1977. Frederick Muller Ltd., London, 1979. Butterfly Books, Australia, 1990.
   Also translated into and published in 7 foriegn languages.

6. *Sai Baba, Invitation to Glory.* Macmillan India Ltd., 1982. Sawbridge Enterprises, London, 1983. Also translated into and published in 2 foreign languages.

7. *The Undiscovered Country.* Sawbridge Enterprises, London, 1984. *Beyond Death: The Undiscovered Country.* Quest Books, Wheaton, U.S.A., 1990.

8. *Where the Road Ends: From Self through Sai to SELF.* Leela Press, U.S.A., 1993.
   Butterfly Books, Australia, 1993. Macmillan India Ltd., India, 1993.

9. *Sai Views and Insights.* Leela Press, U.S.A., 1996. Ganesh & Co., India, 1996.